Better in Bed, No Pills Required

Evidence-Based Natural Solutions for Men's Sexual Health, Stamina & Partner Satisfaction

A Research-Backed Guide with 50+ Scientific Studies

Charles Napoleon Pratt

Table of Contents

Chapter 1: The Modern Sexual Health Crisis...........................1

The Hidden Epidemic 1

Breaking Down the Myths 2

The Science of Sexual Function.......................................4

Your Personal Assessment...5

Chapter 2: The Mind-Body Connection in Sexual Performance
....10

Performance Anxiety 10

Cognitive Restructuring Techniques...............................12

Mindfulness for Sexual Presence 14

Building Sexual Confidence..15

Chapter 3: Physical Foundations Through Targeted Exercise..20

Kegel Mastery for Men 20

Cardiovascular Training for Blood Flow 23

Strength Training for Hormones 25

Yoga and Flexibility Work...27

Key Takeaways...29

Chapter 4: Nutritional Strategies That Actually Work...........31

Foods That Boost Nitric Oxide 31

The Mediterranean Diet Advantage 34

Strategic Supplementation 36

Foods and Habits to Avoid...38

Chapter 5: Sleep, Stress, and Lifestyle Optimization.............42

The Sleep-Testosterone Connection 42

Stress Management Techniques 45

Environmental Detoxification..47

Building Sustainable Habits 50

Chapter 6: Communication and Emotional Intimacy............54

Having the Difficult Conversations 54

Building Emotional Connection......................................57

Addressing Performance Pressure Together 60

Partner Support Strategies...63

Chapter 7: Sensate Focus and Non-Goal Intimacy.................67

Understanding Sensate Focus 67

Stage 1-2: Non-Genital Exploration................................70

Stage 3-4: Including Erogenous Zones 72

Stage 5: Sensual Intercourse..75

Chapter 8: Advanced Techniques for Lasting Longer 81

Understanding Ejaculation Control...................................81

Physical Control Methods...84

Mental Control Strategies 87

Partner Collaboration 91

Chapter 9: Age-Specific Strategies and Adaptations 96

In Your 20s-30s: Prevention and Foundation 96

In Your 40s: The Transition Years 99

In Your 50s-60s: Adaptation and Optimization 103

70s and Beyond: Intimacy Without Limits.....................107

Key Takeaways..110

Chapter 10: Creating Your Personalized Action Plan...........112

Week 1-2: Foundation Building 112

Week 3-4: Momentum Building.....................................115

Month 2-3: Integration and Advancement 119

Long-term Sustainability 123

Troubleshooting Common Challenges 126

Success Metrics and Tracking 130

Resources and Support 133

Your Journey Forward 135

Reference 137

Chapter 1: The Modern Sexual Health Crisis

Sexual health problems have reached epidemic proportions, yet most men suffer in silence. The numbers tell a story that needs to be heard: nearly half of all men will face significant sexual difficulties at some point in their lives. This isn't just about statistics on a page—it's about real men, real relationships, and real suffering that doesn't have to continue.

The good news? You picked up this book, which means you're ready to do something about it. And here's what most doctors won't tell you: the vast majority of sexual health issues can be improved or completely resolved without a single pill. That's right—no prescriptions, no side effects, no dependency. Just proven, natural approaches that address the root causes instead of masking symptoms.

The Hidden Epidemic

Let's start with the hard truth. Erectile dysfunction affects 40% of men over 40, with that percentage climbing to 70% by age 70 (Shamloul & Ghanem, 2013). But here's what's really alarming: we're seeing unprecedented rates in younger men. Recent studies show 8-11% of men in their 20s now report ED, a phenomenon virtually unheard of just two decades ago (Nguyen et al., 2017).

Premature ejaculation? Even more common. Between 30-40% of men struggle with finishing too quickly, making it the most prevalent male sexual dysfunction worldwide (Althof et al., 2014). Think about that—in any room with ten men, three or four are dealing with this issue.

But wait, there's more. (Sorry, had to throw that in there.) Performance anxiety has become so widespread that 60% of young men now report avoiding sexual encounters entirely due to fear of failure (McCabe et al., 2016). They're literally opting out of intimacy because the pressure feels unbearable.

The economic impact? Staggering. Healthcare costs related to sexual dysfunction exceed $146 million annually in the United States alone, and that's just counting men who actually seek help (Goldstein, 2000). Most don't. They suffer quietly, relationships crumble, and the cycle continues.

Here's a real example that might sound familiar. James, a 34-year-old software developer, came to see me after his girlfriend of two years gave him an ultimatum. Their sex life had dwindled from passionate encounters to awkward attempts maybe once a month. He'd started making excuses—too tired, too stressed, had to get up early. Truth was, he'd failed to get an erection three times in a row, and the fear of a fourth failure paralyzed him.

"I lie there at night thinking about it," he told me. "The more I worry, the worse it gets. Now I'm worried about worrying." Sound familiar? James isn't alone. His story plays out in millions of bedrooms across the country.

Breaking Down the Myths

Society has done a spectacular job of screwing up our understanding of male sexuality. We've created myths so powerful they literally cause the problems they claim to describe. Time to bust them wide open.

"Real men don't have problems" might be the most damaging lie we tell. This toxic masculinity garbage suggests that sexual function should be automatic, like breathing. Any deviation from porn-star performance means you're less of a man. Absolute nonsense. Sexual response is complex, involving your cardiovascular system, nervous system, hormones, and psychology all working in concert. Of course things can go sideways sometimes. That's not weakness—that's biology.

Then there's the **pharmaceutical-only myth**—the idea that sexual problems require medical intervention. Don't get me wrong, medications have their place. But natural approaches show improvement rates between 40-73% for erectile dysfunction (Burnett et al., 2018). Many men see complete resolution without ever filling a prescription. The drug companies don't want you to know this, but lifestyle modifications often work better than pills and last longer too.

"Age equals inevitable decline" represents another false belief. Yes, things change as we get older. Recovery time increases, spontaneous erections decrease. But complete sexual dysfunction? Not inevitable. Not even close. I've worked with men in their 70s and 80s who maintain active, satisfying sex lives. The difference? They adapted their approach instead of accepting defeat.

Finally, let's address the **penetration obsession**. Somewhere along the line, we decided that sex equals penis-in-vagina intercourse, period. Everything else became foreplay, secondary, less than. This narrow definition creates massive pressure and ignores the reality that most women don't orgasm from penetration alone anyway (Meston et al., 2004). Expanding our definition of sexual success reduces pressure and increases satisfaction for everyone involved.

Take Robert, a 52-year-old teacher who bought into all these myths. He'd been using ED medication for five years, convinced his age meant natural function was impossible. The pills worked, sort of, but left him with headaches and a stuffy nose. Worse, he felt like a failure for needing them.

We spent six months working on lifestyle changes—exercise, diet, stress management, communication with his wife. Not only did he regain natural function, but their entire relationship transformed. "I wish someone had told me this stuff 20 years ago," he said. "I thought getting older meant giving up. Turns out I just needed to change my approach."

The Science of Sexual Function

Understanding how erections actually work changes everything. Most men have no clue what's happening in their bodies, which makes problems feel mysterious and unfixable. So let's break it down in plain English.

The nitric oxide pathway is your penis's best friend. When you get aroused, your brain sends signals that trigger the release of nitric oxide in penile blood vessels. This causes smooth muscle relaxation, blood flows in, and voilà—erection (Andersson, 2011). Anything that messes with nitric oxide production (smoking, poor diet, lack of exercise) directly impacts your ability to get hard.

But here's where it gets interesting. Your nervous system has two modes: **parasympathetic** (rest and digest) and **sympathetic** (fight or flight). Guess which one you need for sexual function? That's right, parasympathetic. You literally cannot get an erection when your body thinks you're fighting a bear. Yet modern life keeps most of us in constant sympathetic activation—deadlines, traffic, bills, social media. No wonder so many men struggle.

The **hormonal orchestra** adds another layer of complexity. Testosterone gets all the press, but it's actually a symphony of hormones working together. Cortisol (stress hormone) directly suppresses testosterone. Poor sleep tanks growth hormone. Insulin resistance from crappy diet affects everything. These hormones don't exist in isolation—they're constantly influencing each other (Traish, 2014).

Then we have the **brain-body connection**, perhaps the most underappreciated aspect. Your thoughts literally create physical responses. Worry about performance? Your brain interprets that as danger, triggering sympathetic activation and killing any chance of erection. This isn't "all in your head"—it's a real, measurable physiological response.

Let me share Michael's story to illustrate. This 28-year-old came in convinced he had a physical problem. Multiple doctors found nothing wrong. Blood work perfect. Cardiovascular health excellent. Yet he couldn't maintain an erection with partners.

We discovered his problems started after a girlfriend made a cruel comment about his performance during a breakup fight. That single moment created a feedback loop: worry about failure → sympathetic activation → failure → more worry. Once he understood the mechanism, we could interrupt the pattern. Within two months, full function returned.

Your Personal Assessment

Time to get honest about where you stand. No judgment here—just clear-eyed assessment so you know what you're working with.

Start with the **International Index of Erectile Function (IIEF-5)**. This validated questionnaire gives you a baseline score for erectile function (Rosen et al., 1997). Rate the following over the past 6 months:

1. Confidence in getting an erection (1-5 scale)
2. Hardness sufficient for penetration (1-5 scale)
3. Ability to maintain erection (1-5 scale)
4. Difficulty maintaining to completion (1-5 scale)
5. Satisfaction with sexual encounters (1-5 scale)

Score interpretation:

- 22-25: No ED
- 17-21: Mild ED
- 12-16: Mild to moderate ED
- 8-11: Moderate ED
- 5-7: Severe ED

For premature ejaculation, use the **Index of Premature Ejaculation (IPE)** (Althof, 2006). Key questions include:

- Time from penetration to ejaculation
- Control over ejaculation
- Distress level about the problem
- Impact on relationship satisfaction

Now for the crucial part: **identifying your type**. Sexual problems generally fall into three categories:

1. **Primarily physical**: Cardiovascular disease, diabetes, hormonal imbalances, medication side effects
2. **Primarily psychological**: Performance anxiety, depression, relationship issues, past trauma
3. **Mixed**: Most common, involving both physical and psychological factors

Your **risk factor checklist** should include:

Medical factors:

- Cardiovascular disease or risk factors
- Diabetes or prediabetes
- Obesity (BMI over 30)
- Low testosterone symptoms
- Medication use (especially antidepressants, blood pressure meds)
- Sleep apnea
- Chronic health conditions

Lifestyle factors:

- Sedentary behavior (less than 150 minutes exercise weekly)
- Poor diet (high processed foods, low vegetables)
- Smoking or excessive alcohol
- Chronic stress
- Poor sleep (less than 7 hours nightly)
- Pornography overuse

Psychological factors:

- Performance anxiety
- Depression or anxiety disorders
- Relationship problems
- Past sexual trauma
- Body image issues
- Work or financial stress

Setting realistic goals means understanding that improvement takes time. Here's what to expect:

- Week 1-2: Increased awareness, initial habit changes
- Week 3-4: Early physiological improvements (better sleep, less stress)
- Month 2-3: Noticeable changes in function for most men
- Month 3-6: Significant improvement or resolution for 70% of men
- Month 6+: Maintenance and continued optimization

Success isn't just about erections. Track these metrics too:

- Morning erections (frequency and quality)
- Libido level (desire independent of performance)
- Confidence in sexual situations
- Overall relationship satisfaction
- Energy and mood improvements

7

One final assessment tool: the **partner perspective**. If you're in a relationship, their input matters. Often partners notice improvements before you do. They also provide crucial feedback about pressure, expectations, and what really matters to them (hint: it's rarely what you think).

David, a 45-year-old executive, scored 14 on the IIEF-5 (mild to moderate ED) during his initial assessment. He identified multiple risk factors: 60-hour work weeks, poor sleep, pre-diabetes, and zero exercise. His wife Sarah joined our third session and revealed something David hadn't mentioned—their emotional connection had eroded along with their sex life.

"I don't even care about the sex," she said. "I just miss feeling close to him."

This changed our entire approach. Instead of focusing solely on erectile function, we addressed the relationship holistically. Six months later, David's IIEF-5 score hit 23, but more importantly, Sarah reported feeling "like newlyweds again."

Key Takeaways

Sexual dysfunction affects millions of men, but shame keeps most from seeking help. The epidemic is real, growing, and causing massive suffering in relationships worldwide. Young men face unprecedented challenges, with performance anxiety creating a generation afraid of intimacy.

Those toxic myths we've been fed? Pure garbage. Real men absolutely have problems sometimes—it's called being human. Pills aren't the only answer; natural approaches work for most men. Age doesn't doom you to dysfunction, and great sex involves way more than just penetration.

The science shows us that erections require a complex coordination of blood vessels, nerves, hormones, and psychology. Understanding these mechanisms empowers you to address root causes. When you know that stress hormones kill erections, you can do something about stress. When you understand the brain-body connection, you can interrupt negative patterns.

Your honest self-assessment provides the roadmap forward. Whether your issues are primarily physical, psychological, or (most likely) both, identifying specific risk factors allows targeted intervention. Realistic goal-setting prevents discouragement and celebrates small wins along the way.

Most importantly, you're not broken. You're not less of a man. You're someone dealing with a common health issue that has real solutions. The journey ahead requires effort, patience, and probably some uncomfortable conversations. But thousands of men have walked this path successfully, and you can too.

The question isn't whether improvement is possible—research proves it is. The question is whether you're ready to challenge those myths, understand your body, and take action. Based on the fact you're reading this, I'd say you are.

Chapter 2: The Mind-Body Connection in Sexual Performance

Your mind is the most powerful sex organ you have. Forget what you've heard about size or stamina—the six inches between your ears determine what happens with the six inches between your legs. And right now, for millions of men, that mental game is completely broken.

Here's the truth nobody talks about: most sexual dysfunction starts upstairs, not downstairs. Your penis works fine. Your hormones? Probably normal. But that three-pound computer in your skull? It's running outdated software full of bugs, viruses, and malware picked up from years of bad programming. Time for a complete system upgrade.

Performance Anxiety

Performance anxiety is like quicksand—the harder you fight, the deeper you sink. It starts innocently enough. Maybe you had one bad night. Too much to drink, stressed about work, whatever. But then your brain does what brains do best: it creates a story. "What if it happens again?" becomes "It's definitely going to happen again" becomes "I'm broken."

The anxiety-dysfunction cycle works like this: You worry about performance, which triggers your sympathetic nervous system (fight or flight mode). Your body thinks you're being chased by a tiger, so it diverts blood away from "non-essential" functions like erections. You fail to get hard, which confirms your worst fears, creating more anxiety for next time (Bancroft & Janssen, 2000). Round and round we go.

Think about it—have you ever tried to get an erection while doing your taxes? Of course not. Your brain knows the difference between sexy time and stress time. But performance anxiety tricks your body into thinking sex is a high-stakes performance review where your entire worth as a man hangs in the balance.

Cortisol's sabotage makes everything worse. This stress hormone doesn't just kill your mood—it physically blocks the pathways needed for arousal. Studies show that elevated cortisol levels can reduce penile blood flow by up to 70% (McCabe et al., 2016). You might as well try to inflate a balloon with a knot in it.

Then we have **spectatoring syndrome**, first identified by Masters and Johnson in the 1970s. Instead of being in the moment, you float outside your body like a ghost, watching and judging your own performance. "Is it hard enough? Is she enjoying this? Am I taking too long?" You become the world's worst sports commentator for your own sex life.

Marcus, a 31-year-old marketing manager, described it perfectly: "It's like I'm watching myself on a security camera, critiquing every move. The more I watch, the worse I perform. Then I'm watching myself fail, which makes me fail harder." He'd turned sex into a spectator sport where he was simultaneously the player, coach, and harshest critic.

Cultural programming adds another layer of pressure. Movies show men ready for action 24/7. Porn depicts hydraulic penises that stay hard for hours. Social media brags about marathon sessions. We've created impossible standards based on fantasy, then wonder why reality disappoints.

The average man lasts 5-7 minutes during intercourse (Waldinger, 2005). But ask most guys what's "normal," and they'll say 20-30 minutes because that's what culture sells us.

We're literally anxious about not meeting standards that don't exist in nature.

Cognitive Restructuring Techniques

Time to debug that faulty mental software. Cognitive restructuring isn't some new-age nonsense—it's based on decades of research showing that changing thoughts changes outcomes. Your brain believes whatever you tell it repeatedly, so let's start telling it better stories.

Identifying negative thought patterns comes first. Common dysfunctional beliefs include:

- "Real men are always ready"
- "If I can't get hard, I'm not a real man"
- "My partner will leave me if I can't perform"
- "Everyone else has perfect sex lives"
- "One failure means I'm permanently broken"

Sound familiar? These thoughts seem logical in the moment but fall apart under examination. Always ready? Even teenagers have off days. Not a real man? Your worth isn't measured by your erection. Partner will leave? If they'd leave over this, they weren't worth keeping.

The CBT approach challenges these thoughts systematically. When you catch yourself thinking "I'm going to fail again," stop and examine the evidence. How many times have you actually "failed" versus succeeded? What other factors were involved? Would you judge a friend this harshly? (Rosen et al., 2014).

Here's a practical exercise: Write down your worst sexual fear. Now write three pieces of evidence supporting it and three against it. Most men discover their evidence "for" is all assumption and fear, while evidence "against" includes actual facts and experiences.

Reframing success changes the entire game. Instead of "I must maintain a rock-hard erection for 30 minutes," try "I want to connect with my partner and enjoy whatever happens." Success becomes about pleasure, intimacy, and connection—not athletic performance.

Tom, a 38-year-old teacher, transformed his sex life with this simple reframe. "I stopped treating sex like a test I could fail and started treating it like recess—just playing and having fun. Ironically, once I stopped caring about my performance, my performance improved dramatically."

Daily thought exercises cement new patterns:

Morning reframe (5 minutes):

1. Identify one negative sexual thought
2. Challenge it with evidence
3. Create a balanced, realistic alternative
4. Repeat the new thought three times
5. Visualize yourself believing and living it

Evening gratitude practice:

1. Name three things your body did well today (sexual or not)
2. Acknowledge one moment of physical pleasure (eating, stretching, etc.)
3. Thank your body for one specific function
4. Set an intention for tomorrow's physical experience
5. Release any performance pressure for tomorrow

These aren't just feel-good exercises. Neuroplasticity research shows that consistent practice literally rewires your brain, creating new neural pathways that support confidence instead of anxiety (Lutz et al., 2004).

Mindfulness for Sexual Presence

Jon Kabat-Zinn didn't invent mindfulness for better erections, but damn if it doesn't work perfectly for that. Being present during sex sounds obvious—where else would you be? But most men are everywhere except in their bodies during intimate moments.

Present-moment awareness in intimacy means noticing what's actually happening instead of what might happen. Feel the warmth of skin contact. Notice your breathing. Pay attention to sounds, smells, sensations. When your mind wanders to performance worries, gently bring it back to right now.

This isn't mystical—it's practical. When you're fully present, there's no room for anxiety about future performance. You can't worry about keeping an erection while truly focusing on how your partner's breath feels on your neck.

The sensory focus technique grounds you in physical reality:

- **Touch**: Temperature, texture, pressure, movement
- **Sound**: Breathing, heartbeats, voices, ambient noise
- **Sight**: Your partner's expressions, body movements, environment
- **Smell**: Natural scents, perfume, the unique smell of arousal
- **Taste**: Skin, lips, whatever you're experiencing

Practice this during non-sexual touch first. Hold your partner's hand and spend two minutes noticing everything about that contact. Build the skill when stakes are low, then apply it during intimacy.

Non-judgmental observation might be the hardest part. Your penis starts to soften? Notice it without adding commentary. "Oh, I'm getting softer" versus "Oh no, I'm failing again!" See

14

the difference? One is observation, the other is catastrophizing (Stephenson & Kerth, 2017).

James practiced this for weeks before seeing results. "At first, I'd notice my erection fading and panic. But I kept practicing just noticing without judging. 'Huh, getting softer. Interesting. Now it's getting harder again. Cool.' Once I stopped making it mean anything, the fluctuations stopped bothering me."

Partner mindfulness exercises double the benefits:

Synchronized breathing (10 minutes):

1. Lie facing each other, clothed, one hand on partner's chest
2. Feel their breathing rhythm
3. Gradually sync your breathing with theirs
4. Notice without trying to change anything
5. If minds wander, return to breath awareness

Eye gazing (5 minutes):

1. Sit comfortably facing each other
2. Look into one eye (switching is distracting)
3. Notice urges to look away or laugh
4. Stay present with whatever arises
5. No talking—let eyes communicate

These exercises build intimacy while teaching presence. Can't maintain eye contact for five minutes? You're definitely not present during sex.

Building Sexual Confidence

Confidence isn't about believing you're perfect—it's about knowing you can handle imperfection. Sexual confidence means trusting yourself to respond appropriately whatever happens, not guaranteeing specific outcomes.

Visualization techniques train your brain for success. Athletes use this constantly because mental rehearsal activates the same neural pathways as physical practice. Spend five minutes daily visualizing successful intimate encounters—not porn fantasies, but realistic, achievable experiences.

Key visualization elements:

- Start with non-sexual affection
- Include normal variations (sometimes harder, sometimes softer)
- Focus on pleasure and connection, not performance
- Visualize handling challenges calmly
- End with satisfaction regardless of specific acts

Positive self-talk strategies replace that critical inner voice. Instead of "Don't screw this up," try "I'm going to enjoy connecting with my partner." Replace "What if I fail?" with "What if I succeed?" Not fake positivity—realistic encouragement.

Create a personal manifesto:

- "My worth isn't measured by my erection"
- "Sex is about pleasure, not performance"
- "I can satisfy my partner many ways"
- "Every experience teaches me something"
- "I trust my body's wisdom"

Write these down. Say them aloud. Repeat until they feel true. Your brain can't distinguish between what's real and what's vividly imagined and repeated (Cascio et al., 2016).

Body image reconstruction shifts focus from appearance to function. That slight belly? It's powered you through life. Those imperfect muscles? They've carried you everywhere you've been. Your penis? It's brought you pleasure and connection, regardless of size.

List five things your body does well (non-sexual):

1. Carries you through daily life
2. Heals from injuries
3. Experiences pleasure from food
4. Allows you to hug loved ones
5. Keeps functioning despite neglect

Now five sexual functions worth appreciating:

1. Responds to attraction
2. Experiences pleasure
3. Connects with another person
4. Provides stress relief
5. Creates intimacy

Achievement anchoring builds on existing successes. You've had good sexual experiences before—even if anxiety makes them hard to access. Write down three of your best sexual memories. What made them good? Probably not your erection quality but the connection, fun, or intimacy.

Reference these anchors when doubt creeps in. "I've done this successfully before" carries more weight than "I hope I can do this."

David used this technique brilliantly: "I made a mental highlight reel of my best moments—not pornographic, just times I felt confident and connected. Before intimacy, I'd replay one good memory. It reminded my body that it knows what to do."

The goal isn't becoming some sexual superman. It's recognizing you're already enough. Your body works. Your mind can support instead of sabotage. You just need practice using these tools until they become automatic.

One client summed it up perfectly: "I spent years trying to fix my penis when the problem was my thinking. Once I fixed that, everything else followed." He's right. Your mind created this problem, and your mind can solve it.

Key Takeaways

Performance anxiety creates a vicious cycle where fear of failure causes the failure you fear. But this cycle can be broken. The same mind that creates anxiety can create confidence—you just need the right tools and consistent practice.

Cognitive restructuring isn't about positive thinking—it's about accurate thinking. Those catastrophic thoughts about what failure means? They're based on cultural programming, not reality. Challenge them systematically and they lose their power.

Mindfulness brings you back to what's actually happening instead of what might happen. You can't be anxious about future performance while fully experiencing present pleasure. Simple exercises like sensory focus and synchronized breathing build this skill.

Confidence comes from knowing you can handle whatever happens, not from guaranteeing specific outcomes. Visualization, positive self-talk, and achievement anchoring train your brain for success while accepting normal variations.

The mind-body connection works both ways. Yes, mental stress causes physical problems. But mental training creates physical improvements. Every technique in this section has helped thousands of men reclaim their sexual confidence.

Your brain is remarkably plastic—it can rewire itself at any age. Those anxiety patterns took years to develop, but they can be changed in weeks or months with consistent practice. Not overnight, but faster than you think.

Most importantly, you're not broken. You're a normal man dealing with abnormal cultural pressures using outdated mental software. Time to upgrade your thinking, which upgrades everything else.

Chapter 3: Physical Foundations Through Targeted Exercise

Movement is medicine, especially for your penis. While everyone's obsessing over pills and quick fixes, the real secret to sexual vitality has been hiding in plain sight: your body already knows how to heal itself. You just need to show it how.

Exercise isn't just about looking good naked (though that's a nice bonus). It's about creating the physical conditions for optimal sexual function. Better blood flow, balanced hormones, stronger pelvic muscles, reduced stress—exercise delivers all of this without a single side effect. Well, except maybe some sore muscles and the annoying need to do more laundry.

Kegel Mastery for Men

Yes, men have pelvic floor muscles. No, they're not just for women who've had babies. And yes, strengthening them can literally change your sex life. But most men doing Kegels are doing them wrong, which is like going to the gym and lifting imaginary weights.

Finding the right muscles requires more precision than "squeeze like you're stopping pee." The bulbocavernosus muscle wraps around the base of your penis and helps pump blood during erections. The pubococcygeus forms a hammock supporting your pelvic organs. The iliococcygeus and puborectalis complete the team (Stafford et al., 2016). Together, they're your erection's best friends.

Here's the foolproof way to find them: Next time you're urinating, stop mid-stream. Feel that squeeze? That's part of it.

Now, without using your glutes or abs, try to lift your testicles slightly. Different sensation, right? Finally, imagine trying to stop yourself from passing gas. That engages the back portion. All three movements together = your complete pelvic floor.

Progressive training protocol builds strength systematically:

Week 1-2: Foundation

- 10 quick squeezes (1 second each)
- 10 slow holds (3 seconds each)
- 3 times daily
- Focus on isolation (no butt or ab clenching)

Week 3-4: Building Endurance

- 15 quick squeezes
- 10 holds (5 seconds each)
- Add 10 "elevator" exercises (gradual squeeze up, gradual release down)
- 3 times daily

Week 5-8: Power Development

- 20 quick squeezes
- 15 holds (8-10 seconds each)
- 15 elevator exercises
- Add resistance: squeeze against gentle finger pressure on perineum
- 3-4 times daily

Fast-twitch vs slow-twitch training matters because you need both. Fast-twitch fibers create powerful quick contractions (think ejaculation control). Slow-twitch maintain steady tone (think lasting power). Quick pulses train fast-twitch. Long holds build slow-twitch endurance.

21

Advanced variations:

- Standing Kegels (gravity adds resistance)
- Kegels during planks (compound challenge)
- Kegels with breath holds (increases intensity)
- Bridge position Kegels (mimics sexual positions)

Integration techniques make this sustainable. Nobody wants to schedule "Kegel time" forever. Link them to existing habits:

- Red lights = 10 quick squeezes
- Brushing teeth = long holds
- Commercial breaks = elevator exercises
- Waiting in lines = stealth training
- Morning shower = full routine

The beauty? Complete invisibility. You could be doing them right now and nobody would know. (Are you? Good.)

Expected timeline varies, but research shows remarkable consistency. 40% of men with ED see normal function return within 3 months of consistent pelvic floor training (Dorey et al., 2005). Another 35% see significant improvement. That's a 75% success rate from exercises you can do while watching Netflix.

Marcus, a 44-year-old accountant, came to me after his doctor suggested medication. "I don't want to depend on pills," he said. We started basic Kegels. Week one: "I feel silly." Week three: "I think something's happening." Week eight: "Morning erections are back!" Week twelve: "Better than I was at 30."

Common mistakes to avoid:

- Overdoing it (muscles need recovery)
- Holding breath (creates unwanted tension)
- Engaging wrong muscles (glutes/abs compensating)
- Expecting overnight results (this is training, not magic)

- Stopping once improvement starts (maintenance matters)

Cardiovascular Training for Blood Flow

Your penis is basically a specialized blood vessel. Anything good for your heart is good for your erection. But here's what most doctors won't tell you: the specific type, duration, and intensity of cardio makes a massive difference.

The 40-minute prescription isn't arbitrary. Research shows 40 minutes of moderate aerobic exercise, 4 times weekly, improves erectile function equivalent to Viagra in many men (Silva et al., 2017). Less than 30 minutes? Limited benefits. More than 60? Diminishing returns. That 40-minute sweet spot maximizes nitric oxide production and endothelial function.

But what counts as "moderate"? Here's where **heart rate zones** become crucial:

- Zone 2 (60-70% max heart rate): Fat burning, recovery
- Zone 3 (70-80% max heart rate): Aerobic improvement, erectile function sweet spot
- Zone 4 (80-90% max heart rate): Performance training
- Zone 5 (90-100% max heart rate): Maximum effort

For sexual health, Zone 3 is gold. Calculate it: 220 minus your age = max heart rate. Multiply by 0.7-0.8. A 40-year-old? Aim for 126-144 beats per minute.

Best activities ranked by effectiveness:

1. Brisk walking (accessible, sustainable, proven effective)
2. Swimming (full-body, low-impact, excellent circulation)
3. Cycling (targets legs and pelvic region, but watch the seat)
4. Jogging (efficient, but higher injury risk)
5. Rowing (phenomenal full-body option)

6. Dancing (fun, sustainable, partner activity)

Walking deserves special mention. Men who walk briskly for 30-40 minutes daily have 50% lower ED risk than sedentary men (Bacon et al., 2003). It's free, requires no equipment, and you can do it anywhere. Start there.

HIIT protocols offer time-efficient alternatives. High-Intensity Interval Training creates similar vascular benefits in less time:

7-Minute Sexual Health HIIT:

- 30 seconds jumping jacks
- 30 seconds rest
- 30 seconds burpees
- 30 seconds rest
- 30 seconds mountain climbers
- 30 seconds rest
- 30 seconds squat jumps
- 30 seconds rest
- Repeat 2-3 rounds

Studies show even 7-minute daily HIIT sessions improve erectile function markers within 6 weeks (Khoo et al., 2013). Perfect for busy guys who "don't have time" for exercise.

Progressive cardio program:

- Week 1-2: 20 minutes walking, 3x/week
- Week 3-4: 30 minutes brisk walking, 4x/week
- Week 5-6: 35 minutes with hills/intervals, 4x/week
- Week 7-8: 40 minutes mixing walking/jogging, 4x/week
- Week 9+: Maintain 40 minutes, 4x/week, varying activities

Robert, 52, hated exercise. "I'm not a gym guy," he insisted. We started with evening walks with his wife. Just talking,

connecting, moving. Six weeks later: "I feel 10 years younger."
His wife reported... other improvements too. Sometimes the
simplest solutions work best.

Strength Training for Hormones

Cardio helps blood flow, but strength training optimizes
hormones. Specifically, compound movements trigger
testosterone release that no supplement can match. But most
guys waste time on bicep curls when they should focus on
movements that actually move the needle.

Compound movements rule for hormone optimization:

1. Squats (the king of testosterone boosters)
2. Deadlifts (total body hormone activation)
3. Bench press (upper body compound)
4. Pull-ups/rows (back and biceps together)
5. Overhead press (shoulders and core)

Why these? They use multiple large muscle groups
simultaneously, creating maximum metabolic stress and
hormone response. Leg exercises especially boost testosterone—
your quads and glutes are your biggest muscles (Kraemer &
Ratamess, 2005).

Optimal rep ranges balance muscle growth with hormone
production:

- 4-6 reps: Maximum strength, high testosterone spike
- 8-12 reps: Muscle growth, sustained hormone elevation
- 15-20 reps: Endurance, minimal hormone impact

For sexual health, alternate between 4-6 rep heavy days and 8-12
rep moderate days. This maximizes both acute testosterone
spikes and growth hormone release.

Sample hormone-optimizing workout: Monday (Heavy):

- Squats: 4 sets x 5 reps
- Bench press: 4 sets x 5 reps
- Bent-over rows: 4 sets x 6 reps
- Planks: 3 sets x 45 seconds

Thursday (Moderate):

- Deadlifts: 3 sets x 8 reps
- Overhead press: 3 sets x 10 reps
- Pull-ups: 3 sets x 8-12 reps
- Walking lunges: 3 sets x 12 each leg

Recovery importance can't be overstated. Overtraining crashes testosterone faster than a bad breakup. Signs you're overdoing it:

- Decreased morning erections
- Irritability and mood swings
- Disrupted sleep
- Declining performance
- Loss of motivation

Rest days aren't lazy—they're when your body actually builds testosterone. Aim for 2-3 strength sessions weekly, never consecutive days.

Age-specific modifications keep you safe while effective:

- 20s-30s: Full intensity, focus on building base
- 40s: Longer warm-ups, slightly higher reps
- 50s: Extended recovery, emphasis on form
- 60s+: Lower impact variations, machines acceptable
- 70s+: Resistance bands, bodyweight, careful progression

Frank, 58, hadn't lifted since high school. "I don't want to get hurt," he worried. We started with bodyweight squats and modified push-ups. Three months later, he was deadlifting his bodyweight. "My wife says I look like I did at 40," he beamed. More importantly, everything else was working like he was 40 too.

Yoga and Flexibility Work

Before you skip this section because "yoga's for women," consider this: yoga improves erectile function through multiple mechanisms—increased blood flow, reduced stress, better body awareness, and enhanced flexibility for... various positions. Plus, yoga class gender ratios aren't bad either. Just saying.

Five essential poses target sexual health specifically:

1. Cobra Pose (Bhujangasana):
   - Strengthens pelvic muscles
   - Improves spinal flexibility
   - Stimulates abdominal organs
   - Hold 30 seconds, 3 repetitions
2. Bow Pose (Dhanurasana):
   - Intense pelvic floor activation
   - Opens hip flexors
   - Stimulates reproductive organs
   - Hold 20 seconds, 3 repetitions
3. Bridge Pose (Setu Bandhasana):
   - Direct pelvic floor strengthening
   - Improves pelvic tilt
   - Enhances thrust capacity
   - Hold 45 seconds, 3 repetitions
4. Forward Bend (Paschimottanasana):
   - Increases pelvic blood flow
   - Stretches entire posterior chain
   - Calms nervous system
   - Hold 60 seconds, 2 repetitions
5. Child's Pose (Balasana):
   - Complete relaxation

- Reduces cortisol
- Gentle hip opening
- Hold 2-3 minutes

Pelvic floor integration during yoga multiplies benefits. Add gentle Kegel contractions during poses:

- Cobra: Contract on the lift
- Bridge: Hold contraction throughout
- Forward bend: Pulse contractions with breath
- Child's pose: Complete relaxation

Breathing coordination transforms stretching into meditation:

- Inhale 4 counts through nose
- Hold 4 counts
- Exhale 6 counts through mouth
- Pause 2 counts
- Repeat throughout poses

This pranayama (breath control) activates parasympathetic nervous system, essential for arousal.

Partner yoga options build intimacy while improving flexibility:

Seated Spinal Twist:

- Sit back-to-back, legs crossed
- Both twist right, using partner's knee for gentle assistance
- Hold 30 seconds, switch sides
- Synchronize breathing

Partner Forward Fold:

- Sit facing, legs extended, feet touching

- Hold hands/wrists
- Alternate gentle pulling forward
- Creates trust and connection

Double Downward Dog:

- One partner in down-dog
- Other places hands on partner's lower back
- Top partner walks feet up to L-shape
- Builds playfulness and trust

Morning yoga routine (15 minutes):

1. Cat-cow stretches: 10 rounds
2. Cobra pose: 3 holds
3. Bridge pose: 3 holds
4. Forward bend: 2 holds
5. Spinal twists: each side
6. Child's pose: 3 minutes
7. Corpse pose with Kegels: 5 minutes

David, initially skeptical, tried yoga after his wife's suggestion. "I felt ridiculous at first," he admitted. But after six weeks: "I'm more flexible everywhere, if you know what I mean. And the stress relief? Game-changer." His wife enthusiastically confirmed the improvements.

Key Takeaways

Exercise is the closest thing we have to a fountain of youth for sexual function. But not just any movement—targeted, specific protocols that address the root causes of dysfunction.

Kegels aren't just for women. These invisible exercises strengthen the exact muscles responsible for erection quality and ejaculatory control. With proper technique and progression, 75%

of men see significant improvement. No equipment, no gym, no excuses.

Cardiovascular exercise is non-negotiable. That 40-minute prescription isn't arbitrary—it's the proven sweet spot for vascular health. Walking counts. Dancing counts. Find something sustainable and stick with it.

Strength training does more than build muscle. The right exercises trigger hormone cascades that no supplement can match. Focus on compound movements, respect recovery, and watch your body rediscover its vitality.

Yoga might seem unexpected, but the combination of flexibility, strength, breath work, and stress reduction creates powerful sexual health benefits. Plus, partner yoga builds intimacy while building flexibility.

The best program? The one you'll actually do. Start where you are, progress gradually, and stay consistent. Your body wants to function optimally—you just need to create the conditions.

Movement is medicine. Take your dose daily.

Chapter 4: Nutritional Strategies That Actually Work

Food is sexual fuel. But somewhere between fad diets and conflicting nutrition advice, we've forgotten a simple truth: what you eat directly determines how well your penis works. Not metaphorically. Not theoretically. Literally.

Every erection starts with nitric oxide. Every hormone needs raw materials. Every nerve signal requires specific nutrients. You can exercise perfectly, manage stress brilliantly, and communicate like a relationship guru—but if you're eating garbage, you're fighting with one hand tied behind your back. Or more accurately, one blood vessel constricted in your pants.

Foods That Boost Nitric Oxide

Nitric oxide (NO) is your erection's best friend. This molecule relaxes blood vessels, allowing them to expand and fill with blood. No nitric oxide? No erection. It's that simple. Fortunately, certain foods boost NO production naturally, without side effects, and they taste a hell of a lot better than little blue pills.

The beet protocol stands out as the single most powerful dietary intervention. Research shows 70mL of beetroot juice daily increases nitric oxide levels by 21% within hours (Kapil et al., 2015). That's not a typo—21% from drinking less than three ounces of juice.

Here's why beets work: They're loaded with dietary nitrates, which your body converts to nitric oxide through a fascinating process involving your saliva (yes, really). The nitrates become nitrites in your mouth, then NO in your stomach. Nature's chemistry set, right in your kitchen.

Practical beet protocol:

- Morning: 70mL beetroot juice on empty stomach
- Alternative: 1 medium beet, roasted or juiced
- Timing: 2-3 hours before intimate encounters for acute effects
- Daily consumption for chronic benefits
- Mix with apple or carrot juice if taste is challenging

Dark chocolate dosing offers another delicious NO boost. But we're talking real chocolate here—70% cocoa minimum, not that sugary milk chocolate nonsense. Dark chocolate contains flavonoids that stimulate nitric oxide production and improve endothelial function (the lining of your blood vessels).

Optimal protocol:

- 30-40g daily (about 1.5 ounces)
- 70% cocoa or higher
- Consume 1-2 hours before activity for acute benefits
- Split into two servings for better absorption
- Look for low-sugar varieties

Studies show regular dark chocolate consumption improves erectile function scores by 9-16% over 8 weeks (West et al., 2014). Plus, it tastes good and makes you look sophisticated. Win-win.

Watermelon juice benefits come from L-citrulline, an amino acid that converts to L-arginine, which then produces nitric oxide. It's like a natural Viagra growing in your garden. The highest concentrations are in the white rind, so don't throw that away.

Watermelon protocol:

- 16-20 ounces fresh watermelon juice daily

32

- Include some white rind for maximum citrulline
- Best consumed on empty stomach
- Can concentrate by simmering to reduce volume
- Effects build over 3-4 weeks

One study found men drinking watermelon juice reported harder erections and increased satisfaction after just three weeks (Cormio et al., 2011). Summer never sounded so good.

Creating NO-boosting meals throughout the day maintains steady levels:

Breakfast Power Bowl:

- 1 cup oatmeal (contains L-arginine)
- 1 tbsp ground flax seeds (omega-3s)
- Handful of walnuts (more L-arginine)
- Dark berries (antioxidants protect NO)
- Drizzle of honey (natural energy)

Lunch Circulation Salad:

- Mixed dark leafy greens (nitrates)
- Roasted beets (NO superstar)
- Avocado (healthy fats for hormone production)
- Pumpkin seeds (zinc for testosterone)
- Olive oil vinaigrette (more on this soon)

Dinner Performance Plate:

- Wild-caught salmon (omega-3s, vitamin D)
- Roasted garlic (allicin for blood flow)
- Spinach sautéed in olive oil (nitrates + healthy fat)
- Dark chocolate square for dessert

Michael, a 46-year-old chef, laughed when I suggested dietary changes. "I cook for a living—I know food." But his diet was all refined, restaurant-style richness. We shifted to NO-focused meals. Six weeks later: "I feel like I'm 25 again. Who knew beets were better than the pills my doctor offered?"

The Mediterranean Diet Advantage

Forget every fad diet you've heard about. The Mediterranean diet doesn't just help you live longer—it makes those extra years a lot more fun. Research shows men following Mediterranean principles have 65-72% lower risk of ED compared to Western diet followers (Esposito et al., 2010).

Why? This isn't really a "diet"—it's an anti-inflammatory, blood vessel-protecting way of eating that humans thrived on for millennia. Every component supports sexual function through multiple mechanisms.

How olive oil beats Viagra might sound like clickbait, but the science is solid. Nine tablespoons of olive oil weekly improved erectile function more than Viagra in one head-to-head study (Konstantinidis et al., 2019). Not a typo. Olive oil. Beating medication.

The magic comes from:

- Monounsaturated fats that improve cholesterol ratios
- Polyphenols that protect blood vessels
- Anti-inflammatory compounds that reduce ED risk
- Vitamin E for hormone production

Weekly meal planning Mediterranean-style:

- 9 tablespoons extra virgin olive oil (daily drizzle on everything)
- 13+ servings vegetables (almost 2 per day)
- 4 servings legumes (beans, lentils)
- 3 servings fatty fish (salmon, sardines, mackerel)

- 3 servings nuts (walnuts, almonds)
- 2 servings whole grains daily
- 1-2 glasses red wine (optional, has pros and cons)
- Minimal red meat (once weekly max)
- Zero processed foods

This isn't about perfection. It's about shifting your overall pattern toward foods that support rather than sabotage sexual function.

Anti-inflammatory effects protect blood vessels long-term. Chronic inflammation damages the endothelium (blood vessel lining), making erections difficult or impossible. The Mediterranean diet reduces inflammatory markers by 20-40% within weeks (Estruch et al., 2013).

Think of inflammation like rust in your pipes. You can force water through rusty pipes with enough pressure (medication), or you can prevent the rust in the first place (diet). Which sounds smarter?

Age-specific adaptations optimize benefits:

20s-30s: Foundation Building

- Focus on establishing healthy patterns
- Higher calorie needs support more whole grains
- Emphasize antioxidants for prevention

40s-50s: Damage Control

- Increase omega-3 intake
- More aggressive anti-inflammatory foods
- Consider intermittent fasting addition

60s+: Optimization

- Smaller portions, nutrient density matters more

- Extra focus on B12, D3, omega-3s
- Digestive enzymes may help absorption

Carlos, 52, switched from standard American diet to Mediterranean after his first ED episode. "My wife thought I was having a midlife crisis with all the olive oil and fish. But after two months, she stopped complaining. We both lost weight, my blood pressure dropped, and... let's just say she's very happy with the other improvements."

Strategic Supplementation

Let me be clear: supplements supplement a good diet, they don't replace it. But certain nutrients are nearly impossible to get in therapeutic doses from food alone. Smart supplementation fills these gaps without breaking the bank or causing side effects.

The foundational four support overall sexual health:

1. **Vitamin D3 (3000-5000 IU daily)**
   - 45% of men with ED are deficient in vitamin D
   - Supports testosterone production
   - Improves endothelial function
   - Take with fatty meal for absorption
   - Get levels tested (aim for 50-70 ng/mL)
2. **Zinc (15-30mg daily)**
   - Essential for testosterone synthesis
   - Supports prostate health
   - Improves sperm quality
   - Take on empty stomach if tolerated
   - Don't exceed 40mg (interferes with copper)
3. **Magnesium (300-400mg daily)**
   - Relaxes blood vessels
   - Improves sleep quality
   - Reduces stress response
   - Glycinate form absorbs best
   - Take before bed for sleep benefits

4. **Omega-3 (1-2g EPA/DHA daily)**
   o Reduces inflammation
   o Improves blood flow
   o Supports hormone production
   o Look for third-party tested brands
   o Refrigerate to prevent rancidity

Performance enhancers provide targeted benefits:

L-arginine (3-5g daily) serves as direct precursor to nitric oxide. Studies show 5g daily improves erectile function in men with mild to moderate ED within 6 weeks (Chen et al., 1999). However, it's not for everyone:

- Best for men under 50
- Less effective with severe ED
- Can reactivate herpes virus
- Take on empty stomach
- Split into 2-3 doses

L-citrulline (1.5g daily) often works better than L-arginine because it bypasses intestinal breakdown. Research shows significant improvements in erection hardness within 30 days (Cormio et al., 2011):

- Converts to L-arginine in kidneys
- Better absorbed than L-arginine
- No herpes concerns
- Can be taken with food
- Pairs well with beet juice

Timing strategies maximize absorption:

- Fat-soluble vitamins (D3, E, K) with fatty meals
- Minerals (zinc, magnesium) away from calcium
- Amino acids (arginine, citrulline) empty stomach
- Omega-3s with meals to prevent fishy burps

- B-vitamins morning for energy

Quality sourcing prevents wasting money on garbage:

- Third-party testing (USP, NSF, ConsumerLab)
- Avoid proprietary blends
- Check expiration dates
- Research the manufacturer
- Start with single ingredients, not complexes
- Buy from reputable sources (not gas stations)

Tom came to me taking 15 different supplements, spending $300 monthly. "My medicine cabinet looks like a health food store," he complained. We streamlined to the foundational four plus citrulline. Not only did he save money, but his results improved. Sometimes less is more.

Foods and Habits to Avoid

Knowing what to eat is only half the equation. Some foods and habits actively sabotage sexual function. Think of them as kryptonite for your penis—avoid them like your sex life depends on it. Because it does.

The testosterone killers hide in plain sight:

Processed foods deliver a triple threat:

- Trans fats damage blood vessels
- High sodium increases blood pressure
- Chemical preservatives disrupt hormones
- Aim for less than 10% calories from processed sources

Excess alcohol seems paradoxical—it lowers inhibitions but kills performance:

- More than 2 drinks acutely impairs erections

- Chronic use lowers testosterone
- Beer especially problematic (hops contain phytoestrogens)
- Red wine in moderation may be exception

High sugar intake creates multiple problems:

- Causes insulin resistance
- Promotes inflammation
- Reduces testosterone
- Damages blood vessels
- Limit added sugars to 25g daily

Environmental toxins deserve special attention. BPA and phthalates, found in plastics and personal care products, act as endocrine disruptors (Swan, 2021):

Common sources to avoid:

- Plastic water bottles (especially if heated)
- Canned foods (BPA in lining)
- Synthetic fragrances
- Non-stick cookware
- Receipts (BPA coating)

Simple swaps:

- Glass or stainless steel water bottles
- Fresh or frozen over canned
- Fragrance-free products
- Cast iron or stainless cookware
- Decline receipts when possible

Timing considerations around intimacy:

- No large meals 2-3 hours before
- Avoid alcohol beyond one drink

- Skip heavy, fatty foods day-of
- Hydrate throughout the day
- Light, energizing snacks are fine

Hydration optimization often gets overlooked:

- Dehydration reduces blood volume
- Aim for half body weight in ounces daily
- More if exercising or hot climate
- Spread throughout day
- Monitor urine color (pale yellow ideal)

Steve, a 41-year-old salesman, couldn't understand his issues. "I eat pretty healthy," he insisted. But his "healthy" included daily diet soda, microwaved plastic containers, and cologne you could smell from space. We eliminated endocrine disruptors and his testosterone increased 35% in three months. Sometimes it's not what you add, but what you remove.

Key Takeaways

Food is medicine, especially for sexual function. Every meal either supports or sabotages your performance. The choice is yours, three times a day.

Nitric oxide boosting foods work as well as medications for many men. Beets, dark chocolate, and watermelon aren't just healthy—they're natural performance enhancers. Creating NO-focused meals throughout the day maintains the vascular health essential for strong erections.

The Mediterranean diet isn't just heart-healthy—it's penis-healthy. That 65% reduction in ED risk isn't theoretical; it's what happens when you eat foods that reduce inflammation, support blood flow, and optimize hormones. Nine tablespoons of olive oil really can outperform pharmaceuticals.

Strategic supplementation fills nutritional gaps that diet alone can't address. The foundational four—D3, zinc, magnesium, and omega-3s—support every aspect of sexual health. Performance enhancers like L-citrulline provide targeted benefits when used correctly.

What you avoid matters as much as what you consume. Processed foods, excess alcohol, and environmental toxins actively sabotage sexual function. Simple swaps and timing strategies minimize their impact.

The best diet is one you'll actually follow. Start with one change—maybe daily beet juice or switching to olive oil. Build from there. Your body wants to function optimally; you just need to give it the right fuel.

Real food. Real results. No prescription required.

Chapter 5: Sleep, Stress, and Lifestyle Optimization

Your body rebuilds itself while you sleep. Your stress levels determine if that rebuilding actually happens. And your daily habits create the environment where sexual health either thrives or dies. Miss any of these three pillars, and you're basically trying to build a house on quicksand.

Most men think sexual health is about what happens in the bedroom. Wrong. It's about what happens in the other 23 hours and 45 minutes of your day. Every choice you make—from when you go to bed to how you handle your boss's ridiculous demands—directly impacts your ability to perform when it matters.

The Sleep-Testosterone Connection

Sleep isn't just rest—it's when your body manufactures the hormones that make you a man. Literally. Skip sleep, and you're chemically castrating yourself. Sound dramatic? The research says otherwise.

The 7-9 hour imperative isn't some arbitrary recommendation from health nuts. Men who sleep less than 7 hours nightly have testosterone levels of someone 10 years older (Leproult & Van Cauter, 2011). One week of sleeping 5 hours per night cuts testosterone by 15%. That's the equivalent of aging a decade in seven days.

Here's what happens hour by hour:

- Hours 1-3: Deep sleep, growth hormone release
- Hours 4-6: REM cycles intensify, testosterone production peaks

- Hours 7-9: Final REM cycles, cortisol regulation

Cut sleep short, and you're literally stopping the assembly line before the product is finished.

REM sleep importance can't be overstated. This is when 90% of your daily testosterone gets produced. REM sleep typically dominates the final third of your night. Go to bed at midnight and wake at 5 AM? You've missed most of your testosterone factory's production window.

The cruel irony? Low testosterone causes sleep problems, which further reduces testosterone. It's like your body's playing a sick joke on itself.

Sleep apnea solutions deserve special attention because this condition destroys both sleep quality and sexual function. Men with untreated sleep apnea have 70% higher rates of ED (Budweiser et al., 2009). Why? Oxygen deprivation during sleep damages blood vessels and crashes testosterone.

Signs you might have sleep apnea:

- Loud snoring (partner complaints)
- Waking gasping or choking
- Morning headaches
- Daytime exhaustion despite "sleeping" 8 hours
- Decreased morning erections

CPAP (Continuous Positive Airway Pressure) therapy improves erectile function in 75% of men with sleep apnea within 3 months. Yes, the mask looks ridiculous. Yes, it takes adjustment. But you know what's more ridiculous? Choosing erectile dysfunction over wearing a mask to bed.

Optimization protocol for maximum hormonal benefit:

Temperature control:

- Bedroom 65-68°F (18-20°C)
- Cooling mattress pad if needed
- Light sheets, heavy blankets (adjustable)
- Feet can stick out (thermal regulation)

Darkness requirements:

- Blackout curtains or eye mask
- No LED lights (tape over them)
- Phone face-down or outside room
- Red light only if needed for bathroom

Timing strategies:

- Consistent bedtime within 30-minute window
- No screens 1 hour before bed
- Last meal 3 hours before sleep
- Morning light exposure within 30 minutes of waking

Sleep stack for difficult cases:

- Magnesium glycinate: 400mg
- L-theanine: 200mg
- Melatonin: 0.5-1mg (less is more)
- Ashwagandha: 600mg
- Take 30-60 minutes before bed

James, a 43-year-old executive, came to me exhausted and frustrated. "I'm in bed 8 hours but feel like crap," he complained. His wife mentioned his snoring sounded "like a freight train." Sleep study revealed severe apnea—he was stopping breathing 47 times per hour.

Three months after starting CPAP: "I feel like I've been living in a fog for years and suddenly can see clearly. Morning erections are back, energy through the roof, and my wife says I'm like a different person in bed." All from fixing his sleep.

Stress Management Techniques

Stress is an erection killer. Not metaphorically—literally. Cortisol, your primary stress hormone, directly opposes testosterone. When cortisol goes up, testosterone goes down. When stress becomes chronic, your penis basically goes on strike.

Cortisol reduction strategies that actually work:

Meditation isn't just for monks:

- 10 minutes daily reduces cortisol by 23%
- Increases testosterone and DHEA
- Improves heart rate variability
- Apps like Headspace or Calm make it simple
- Start with 2 minutes if 10 seems impossible

Exercise timing matters:

- Morning exercise reduces cortisol all day
- Evening intense exercise can disrupt sleep
- 30-minute walk lowers cortisol immediately
- Yoga combines movement with mindfulness
- Sex counts as exercise (convenient, right?)

Time management reduces chronic stress:

- Say no to non-essential commitments
- Batch similar tasks together
- Take actual breaks (not phone scrolling)
- Leave work at work (radical concept)
- Schedule intimate time like important meetings

Breathing exercises provide immediate relief. Your breath directly controls your nervous system. Fast, shallow breathing = stress response. Slow, deep breathing = relaxation response.

Box breathing technique:

1. Inhale 4 counts through nose
2. Hold 4 counts
3. Exhale 4 counts through mouth
4. Hold empty 4 counts
5. Repeat 4-8 cycles

4-7-8 technique for acute anxiety:

1. Exhale completely
2. Inhale through nose 4 counts
3. Hold breath 7 counts
4. Exhale through mouth 8 counts
5. Repeat 3-4 cycles

This literally forces your nervous system into parasympathetic (rest and digest) mode. Can't get an erection in fight-or-flight mode? Switch modes with your breath.

Progressive muscle relaxation releases physical tension:

Quick version (5 minutes):

1. Tense toes for 5 seconds, release
2. Tense calves for 5 seconds, release
3. Continue up body (thighs, glutes, abs, chest, arms, shoulders, neck, face)
4. Notice the contrast between tension and relaxation
5. End with full-body scan for remaining tension

Full version includes visualization and takes 15-20 minutes. Perfect before bed or intimate encounters.

Creating transition rituals shifts you from work mode to life mode:

The problem: You carry work stress into the bedroom. Your body doesn't know the spreadsheet crisis is over. It's still pumping stress hormones when you're trying to get intimate.

Solution rituals:

- Change clothes immediately when home
- 5-minute breathing session in car before entering house
- Hot shower with eucalyptus oil
- 10-minute walk around block
- Phone in drawer for first hour home

Mark, a surgeon, couldn't "turn off" after work. "I'm physically home but mentally still in the OR," he explained. We created a ritual: park in driveway, 4-7-8 breathing five times, visualize putting work in a box, then enter home. "It sounds silly, but it works. My wife noticed immediately. Said I actually seem present now."

Environmental Detoxification

Your environment is loaded with chemical castrators. Sounds like conspiracy theory nonsense, but the science is undeniable. Endocrine disruptors are everywhere, and they're wreaking havoc on male hormones.

Identifying hormone disruptors in your daily life:

BPA (Bisphenol A):

- Plastic water bottles
- Food can linings
- Receipt paper
- Plastic food containers

- Effects: Mimics estrogen, lowers testosterone

Phthalates:

- Personal care products with fragrance
- Vinyl flooring
- Shower curtains
- Air fresheners
- Effects: Reduces sperm quality, disrupts hormones

Parabens:

- Shampoos and body washes
- Deodorants
- Lotions
- Shaving products
- Effects: Estrogenic activity, thyroid disruption

Simple swaps that make a big difference:

Kitchen overhaul:

- Glass containers instead of plastic
- Stainless steel water bottle
- Cast iron or stainless cookware
- Parchment paper instead of plastic wrap
- Ceramic or glass plates (no melamine)

Bathroom detox:

- Fragrance-free products only
- Natural soap (Dr. Bronner's)
- Aluminum-free deodorant
- Coconut oil for moisturizer
- Essential oils instead of cologne

Water and air quality affect hormones more than you'd think:

Water filtration:

- Reverse osmosis or quality carbon filter
- Shower filter (skin absorbs chemicals)
- Glass or stainless for storage
- Avoid bottled water (plastic + sitting = bad)

Air quality:

- HEPA filter in bedroom
- Plants that filter air (snake plant, pothos)
- Open windows when possible
- No synthetic air fresheners
- Regular vacuuming with HEPA vacuum

Creating a sexual health sanctuary in your bedroom:

The bedroom should support two things: sleep and sex. Everything else is a distraction.

Remove:

- Television (kills intimacy)
- Work materials (stress reminders)
- Exercise equipment (except maybe that)
- Clutter (visual stress)
- Bright lights (install dimmers)

Add:

- Blackout curtains
- Quality mattress
- Organic sheets (no pesticides)
- Air purifier
- Red light bulbs for evening
- Lock on door (if kids)

Temperature matters for more than sleep. Cooler temperatures increase testosterone production and make you seek body warmth (hint, hint).

David thought I was crazy when I suggested environmental changes. "What's my deodorant got to do with my erection?" Six weeks after switching to natural products and ditching plastics, his testosterone increased 28%. "I feel like I've been poisoning myself for years," he said. Small changes, big results.

Building Sustainable Habits

Knowledge without action is worthless. You need systems, not willpower. Habits, not heroics. The goal is making healthy choices automatic, not exhausting.

The 21-day protocol leverages neuroplasticity:

Days 1-7: Foundation

- Pick ONE habit to start
- Make it stupidly easy
- Track with simple checkmark
- No exceptions, no excuses
- Celebrate small wins

Days 8-14: Consistency

- Same habit, same time
- Link to existing routine
- Notice resistance patterns
- Push through anyway
- Increase slightly if easy

Days 15-21: Integration

- Habit should feel normal

- Add second habit if ready
- First habit continues
- Notice positive effects
- Plan next progression

Common mistake: Trying to change everything at once. That's not courage, it's stupidity. One habit at a time.

Habit stacking links new behaviors to established routines:

Morning stack:

- Wake up → Drink water (existing)
- Drink water → 10 Kegels (new)
- Kegels → Shower (existing)
- Shower → Cold finish (new)

Evening stack:

- Dinner → Walk (new)
- Walk → Shower (existing)
- Shower → Magnesium (new)
- Magnesium → Read (existing)

The existing habit becomes the trigger for the new one. Your brain already has the neural pathway; you're just adding a detour.

Accountability systems multiply success rates:

Partner involvement:

- Share your goals openly
- Ask for specific support
- Create mutual objectives
- Celebrate together
- Be honest about struggles

Tracking tools:

- Simple calendar X method
- Phone apps (Habitica, Streaks)
- Spreadsheet if you're nerdy
- Physical journal
- Weekly review sessions

Social pressure (positive):

- Tell friends your goals
- Join online community
- Find accountability buddy
- Share progress publicly
- Create consequences for failure

Maintaining motivation when enthusiasm fades:

The honeymoon phase ends. Initial excitement disappears. This is normal and expected. Plan for it.

Motivation sustainers:

- Review your "why" weekly
- Track lead measures, not just outcomes
- Reward milestones (not with food)
- Visualize future self
- Read success stories

When you want to quit:

- Commit to just one more day
- Reduce but don't stop
- Review progress made
- Talk to someone who gets it
- Remember why you started

Richard started strong then crashed week three. "I missed one day and gave up," he admitted. We implemented the "two-day rule"—never miss twice. One miss is life, two is a pattern starting. Six months later, he'd only missed five days total. "That rule saved me. Took the perfectionism pressure off."

Key Takeaways

Sleep is not optional for sexual health. Those 7-9 hours are when your body produces the hormones that make everything else possible. Shortchange sleep, and you're shortchanging your manhood. Literally.

Stress management isn't soft—it's strategic. Chronic stress chemically castrates you through cortisol. Simple techniques like breathing exercises and transition rituals can shift your nervous system in minutes. Your penis works in rest mode, not stress mode.

Your environment is either supporting or sabotaging your hormones. Those convenient plastics and fragranced products? They're convenient testosterone killers. Simple swaps remove the chemical burden and let your body function normally.

Building habits beats relying on willpower every time. The 21-day protocol, habit stacking, and accountability systems turn healthy choices into automatic behaviors. Start small, stay consistent, and let momentum build.

None of this is complicated. Go to bed on time. Manage your stress. Clean up your environment. Build better habits. Your body wants to function optimally—stop getting in its way.

The prescription is simple. The results are profound. The choice is yours.

Chapter 6: Communication and Emotional Intimacy

Sexual problems are relationship problems. Period. You can have perfect blood flow, optimal hormones, and Olympic-level fitness—but if you can't talk to your partner about what's happening between the sheets, you're fighting a losing battle. And here's the kicker: most couples would rather have root canals than honest conversations about sexual struggles.

The silence is deafening. Men suffer alone, convinced they're failures. Partners feel rejected, unwanted, confused. Both sides build walls of assumptions and resentment. Meanwhile, the solution sits right there in the space between you—honest, vulnerable communication. But nobody teaches us how to have these conversations without drowning in shame, blame, and hurt feelings.

Having the Difficult Conversations

Starting a conversation about sexual problems feels like defusing a bomb. Say the wrong thing, and everything explodes. Say nothing, and the problem grows until it explodes anyway. There's no perfect time, no perfect words. But there are ways to make these discussions productive instead of destructive.

Opening scripts that actually work start with ownership, not accusation. The difference between success and disaster often comes down to those first few sentences.

Instead of: "We need to talk about your problem." Try: "I've been struggling with something and could use your support."

Instead of: "You never initiate anymore." Try: "I miss feeling close to you and want to understand what's happening for us."

Instead of: "Our sex life sucks." Try: "I'd love to explore ways we can both feel more satisfied."

See the pattern? You're inviting collaboration, not assigning blame. You're sharing vulnerability, not launching attacks.

Here's a complete opening script that's worked for hundreds of couples:

"I've been thinking about our intimate life, and I realize I haven't been as open as I should be. I've been dealing with some challenges around [specific issue], and I think my silence has created distance between us. I love you and value our connection, and I'd like to share what's been happening for me. Is now a good time, or could we set aside time to talk when we won't be interrupted?"

"I" statements mastery changes everything. They're not just therapy-speak—they're relationship survival tools. "I" statements own your experience without making your partner defensive.

The formula: "I feel [emotion] when [specific situation] because [your need/value]."

Examples:

- "I feel anxious when we're intimate because I worry about disappointing you."
- "I feel disconnected when we don't talk about this because emotional intimacy matters to me."
- "I feel frustrated when I can't perform because I want to please you."

Common mistakes:

- "I feel like you're pressuring me" (hidden "you" statement)
- "I feel that you don't understand" (opinion, not feeling)
- "I feel rejected because you never..." (generalizing)

Active listening techniques ensure both people feel heard. Most of us listen to respond, not to understand. That's like playing tennis while staring at your own racket.

Mirror: Reflect back what you heard

- Partner: "I feel unwanted when you avoid intimacy."
- You: "You're feeling unwanted because I've been avoiding intimacy."
- Not interpretation, just reflection

Validate: Acknowledge their experience

- "That makes sense you'd feel that way."
- "I can understand why that would hurt."
- "Your feelings are completely valid."
- Don't have to agree, just acknowledge

Empathize: Connect emotionally

- "That must be really painful."
- "I imagine that feels lonely."
- "I'd probably feel the same way."
- Feel with them, not for them

Creating safe spaces requires both environmental and emotional preparation. You can't have vulnerable conversations in hostile territory.

Environmental safety:

- Private space (lock doors if kids)

- Phones off and away
- Comfortable seating (side by side often better than face to face)
- Soft lighting (harsh lights increase defensiveness)
- Time buffer (not right before work)
- Tissues available (tears happen)

Emotional safety:

- Agree on ground rules (no yelling, name-calling, threatening)
- Set time limit (30-45 minutes max initially)
- Allow breaks if overwhelmed
- No alcohol (seems helpful but impairs communication)
- Start with appreciation (creates positive foundation)
- End with connection (hug, kind words, future plan)

Michael and Sarah had avoided "the talk" for two years. "Every time we tried, it became a fight," Michael explained. They finally succeeded using this structure: Sunday morning (relaxed time), living room (neutral space), phones in kitchen (no distractions), started by each sharing three things they loved about their relationship (positive foundation). "It was still hard," Sarah said, "but we finally heard each other instead of defending ourselves."

Building Emotional Connection

Sex without emotional connection is just friction. Sure, friction can feel good, but it's not intimacy. Real sexual healing happens when emotional bonds strengthen alongside physical improvements. Most men miss this completely, focusing on hydraulics while ignoring heart stuff.

The four types of intimacy work together like instruments in a band. Miss one, and the whole song sounds off.

Emotional intimacy: Sharing feelings, fears, dreams

- Goes beyond "fine" when asked how you are
- Includes negative emotions, not just positive
- Requires vulnerability and trust
- Built through consistent small shares

Intellectual intimacy: Connecting through ideas

- Discussing books, podcasts, articles
- Sharing opinions respectfully
- Learning together
- Challenging each other's thinking

Physical intimacy: Touch without sexual agenda

- Holding hands during walks
- Massage without expectation
- Cuddling while watching TV
- Dancing in the kitchen

Spiritual intimacy: Shared meaning and values

- Doesn't require religion
- What matters most to both
- Life purpose discussions
- Creating rituals together

Daily connection rituals build intimacy like compound interest—small deposits creating wealth over time (Gottman & Silver, 2015).

Morning check-in (2 minutes):

- "What's on your plate today?"
- "What do you need from me?"
- "What are you looking forward to?"

- Kiss lasting 6+ seconds

Evening gratitude (5 minutes):

- Share one thing you appreciated about partner
- Share one good thing from your day
- Share one challenge you faced
- Physical touch while talking

Weekly deeper dive (20 minutes):

- No phones, full attention
- "What made you feel loved this week?"
- "What was hard for you?"
- "What do you need more/less of?"

Love maps mean knowing your partner's inner world as well as you know your phone apps. Most couples know shockingly little about each other's current reality.

Love map questions:

- Current stressors and worries
- Active hopes and dreams
- Best friend's name
- Favorite way to relax
- Biggest fear right now
- Proudest recent accomplishment
- Childhood memory affecting them
- What they need to feel loved

Update regularly—people change. That favorite movie from dating? Might bore them now. Stay curious.

Vulnerability exercises create deeper connection than years of surface chat (Brown, 2012).

Fear inventory:

1. Each write 3 current fears
2. Share without minimizing
3. No fixing or advice
4. Just witness and acknowledge
5. Find one fear you share

Dream sharing:

1. Describe ideal life in 5 years
2. Include wild, "unrealistic" dreams
3. Partner asks curious questions
4. No judgment or reality checks
5. Find ways to support even small steps

36 questions that lead to love:

- Research-based questions increasing intimacy
- Start surface, go progressively deeper
- Take turns answering
- Maintain eye contact
- End with 4 minutes silent eye gazing

Tom and Lisa felt like roommates after 15 years. "We knew everything about each other," Tom said. Wrong. The love map exercise revealed Lisa had changed careers dreams, Tom had developed new fears about aging, neither knew the other's current struggles. "It was like meeting again," Lisa said. "But better because we had history to build on."

Addressing Performance Pressure Together

Performance pressure doubles when you're trying to succeed for two. Every failed erection feels like failing your partner. Every quick finish seems like selfishness. The weight of their disappointment—real or imagined—crushes any chance of recovery. Time to rewrite the rules together.

Redefining success as a couple means expanding beyond penetration and orgasms. What if success meant:

- Feeling close and connected
- Enjoying physical pleasure (any kind)
- Being vulnerable together
- Laughing during intimate moments
- Exploring without agenda
- Communicating openly
- Taking pressure off

New definitions might include:

- "Success is both of us feeling valued"
- "Success is staying present together"
- "Success is trying something new"
- "Success is honest communication"
- "Success is pleasure without goals"

Create your own definition together. Write it down. Reference it when old pressures creep in.

Creating pressure-free zones gives relief from performance demands:

Designated no-goal times:

- Sunday morning cuddles (no escalation expected)
- Shower together Tuesday/Thursday (just washing)
- Massage Monday (truly just massage)
- Naked Netflix Friday (skin contact, no pressure)

The rules:

- No genital contact unless mutually initiated
- No subtle pressure or hints
- Enjoy what is, not what could be
- If arousal happens, notice without acting
- Build comfort with non-sexual nudity

Stop/slow/go signals prevent misunderstandings during intimacy:

Create your system:

- Green: "Yes, more, keep going"
- Yellow: "Slow down, need adjustment"
- Red: "Stop, need break"

Can be:

- Words ("green," "yellow," "red")
- Touches (squeeze once, twice, three times)
- Sounds (moan, "mmm," silence)
- Movements (pull closer, still, push away)

Practice during non-sexual touch first. Make it automatic before high-stakes moments.

Celebrating effort over outcome rewires success patterns:

What to celebrate:

- Initiating difficult conversation
- Trying new technique
- Staying present during anxiety
- Communicating need or boundary
- Being vulnerable
- Supporting partner
- Not giving up

How to celebrate:

- Verbal appreciation ("I loved how you...")
- Physical affection (type partner prefers)
- Special treats (favorite meal, activity)
- Written notes (text, card, mirror message)
- Quality time (walk, bath, date)

David and Maria created "intimacy wins" jar. Any positive step—from holding hands to honest conversation—earned a note in the jar. Monthly, they'd read them together. "It showed us how much good was happening even when sex wasn't 'working,'" Maria explained. "Took pressure off the bedroom."

Partner Support Strategies

Partners hold tremendous power—to heal or harm. One wrong word during vulnerability can set recovery back months. One right response can accelerate healing beyond belief. Most partners want to help but don't know how. They're scared of making things worse, so they say nothing. Or they try to help in ways that increase pressure.

What to say during difficult moments matters enormously:

When he can't get/maintain erection:

- "I love being close to you."
- "There's no rush, we have all night."
- "Let's just enjoy touching."
- "Your worth isn't measured by your erection."
- "I'm happy just being here with you."

When he finishes quickly:

- "I love that I excite you."
- "We can always go for round two."

- "There are so many ways to pleasure me."
- "That felt good, now let's focus on me."
- "I enjoy our connection regardless."

When he's anxious/worried:

- "We're a team, we'll figure this out."
- "Your vulnerability is attractive."
- "I'm not going anywhere."
- "What would feel good right now?"
- "Let's take the pressure off."

What not to say (even if thinking it):

- "Is it me?" (makes it about you)
- "This never happened with my ex" (comparison kills)
- "Just relax" (if he could, he would)
- "Maybe you should see a doctor" (during the moment)
- "Are you gay?" (orientation isn't the issue)
- "I guess we're done" (fatalistic)
- Silent disappointment (speaks louder than words)

Being an active participant means more than just avoiding harm:

Learn together:

- Read this book as couple
- Watch educational videos
- Attend workshop or therapy
- Practice exercises together
- Share what you learn

Participate in solutions:

- Join exercise routines
- Cook healthy meals together

- Practice stress reduction
- Do Kegel exercises too
- Create sleep sanctuary

Initiate differently:

- Remove penetration expectation
- Start with massage
- Use more words, less groping
- Build anticipation throughout day
- Focus on his pleasure sometimes

Managing your own anxieties prevents emotional contagion (Hatfield et al., 1994):

Common partner anxieties:

- "Is it my fault?"
- "Am I not attractive?"
- "Will this ever improve?"
- "Should I leave?"
- "Am I being too patient?"

Self-care essentials:

- Individual therapy or support group
- Maintain own friendships
- Continue personal hobbies
- Exercise for stress relief
- Journal feelings privately
- Set boundaries kindly

Jennifer struggled when Mark's ED began. "I made it all about me—my attractiveness, my worth, my needs." Her therapist helped her separate her self-worth from his erection. "Once I stopped taking it personally, I could actually support him. Ironically, that's when things improved."

Key Takeaways

Communication about sexual problems requires courage, skill, and practice. But silence guarantees suffering while honest conversation opens doors to healing. Those first conversations feel impossibly hard until you realize the alternative—growing distance and resentment—is harder.

Emotional intimacy isn't optional for sexual healing. The four types of intimacy work together, creating a foundation strong enough to weather any sexual storm. Daily rituals build connection incrementally. Love maps keep you current with your evolving partner. Vulnerability exercises deepen bonds beyond what you thought possible.

Redefining success as a couple removes the win/lose dynamic from sex. When pleasure, connection, and communication become the goals, pressure evaporates. Creating pressure-free zones gives space to just be together. Clear signals prevent misunderstandings. Celebrating effort rewires your definition of success.

Partners can accelerate healing or accidentally sabotage it. Knowing what to say—and what never to say—during vulnerable moments makes all the difference. Active participation means joining the journey, not just watching from sidelines. Managing your own anxieties prevents them from infecting the relationship.

The path forward requires both people. Sexual problems affect relationships, but relationships can also heal sexual problems. When two people commit to honest communication, emotional intimacy, and mutual support, what seemed impossible becomes inevitable.

Connection first. Everything else follows

Chapter 7: Sensate Focus and Non-Goal Intimacy

Sex has become a performance. We've turned the most natural human connection into an Olympic event with judges, scores, and medal ceremonies. No wonder so many men freeze up when the starting gun fires. But what if I told you the secret to mind-blowing sex is to stop trying to have sex at all?

Masters and Johnson figured this out in the 1960s, and their discovery remains the gold standard for treating sexual dysfunction without pills. They called it sensate focus—basically, touching without goals. Sounds simple. Feels revolutionary. Because when you remove the pressure to perform, something magical happens: your body remembers how to respond naturally.

Understanding Sensate Focus

Sensate focus isn't some hippie nonsense about tantric energy. It's a scientifically validated technique that rewires your sexual response by removing the very thing that's breaking it—performance pressure. Think of it as physical therapy for your sex life.

Masters and Johnson's legacy began when they noticed something counterintuitive: the harder couples tried to fix sexual problems, the worse things got. Like quicksand—struggling makes you sink faster. So they created exercises that banned the very outcomes people desperately wanted (Masters & Johnson, 1970).

No orgasms allowed. No penetration permitted. Just... touch.

The genius lies in the paradox. By removing goals, you remove failure. Can't fail at having an orgasm if orgasm isn't allowed. Can't disappoint with a soft erection if erections aren't the point. Suddenly, touch becomes about pleasure, not performance.

Why it works comes down to basic psychology and physiology:

1. Eliminates spectatoring (watching yourself perform)
2. Activates parasympathetic nervous system (rest and arousal)
3. Builds new neural pathways (pleasure without pressure)
4. Increases body awareness (feeling instead of thinking)
5. Reduces anticipatory anxiety (nothing to anticipate)
6. Strengthens couple bond (shared vulnerability)

The research backs this up consistently. Studies show 70-80% improvement rates for various sexual dysfunctions using sensate focus (McCarthy & Wald, 2013). That's better than most medications, with zero side effects except maybe more intimacy than you can handle.

Common mistakes that sabotage success:

Hidden agendas: "I'll pretend there's no goal, but really I'm hoping..."

- Your body knows when you're lying
- Partners sense the pressure
- Defeats entire purpose
- Stay honest about intentions

Rushing stages: "We did stage 1 for ten minutes, ready for intercourse!"

- Each stage needs multiple sessions
- Some couples spend weeks per stage
- Rushing guarantees failure

- Trust the process

Treating it mechanically: "Touch here for 5 minutes, then there for 5..."

- This isn't a recipe
- Stay curious and exploratory
- Let sensation guide you
- Quality over checkboxes

Avoiding difficult feelings: "I felt anxious so we stopped"

- Anxiety is expected
- Notice without escaping
- Breathe through discomfort
- Growth lives in discomfort

Success statistics tell the real story:

- 75% of men with ED show improvement
- 80% of premature ejaculation cases improve
- 68% of low desire issues resolve
- 90% report better relationship satisfaction
- Results maintain long-term (Weiner & Constance, 2017)

But here's what statistics don't capture: the profound shift in how couples relate. When performance pressure lifts, playfulness returns. When touching becomes exploring instead of achieving, wonder replaces worry.

Robert and Janet, married 18 years, hadn't touched beyond perfunctory pecks in three years. "Sex became this thing we failed at," Robert explained. Six weeks of sensate focus later: "We giggle like teenagers. Last night we spent an hour just exploring each other's backs. Who knew shoulder blades could be erotic?"

Stage 1-2: Non-Genital Exploration

Starting with non-genital touch feels like going backwards. You want to fix sexual problems by avoiding sexual areas? Exactly. That's the brilliant misdirection that makes it work. Your genitals have become associated with pressure and failure. Time to remind your body that pleasure exists everywhere.

Setting up sessions requires more thought than "let's get naked and see what happens."

Environmental preparation:

- Warm room (cold kills relaxation)
- Soft lighting (candles or lamps)
- Clean sheets (fresh sensation)
- Door locked (zero interruption worry)
- Phones off AND in another room
- 30-45 minutes minimum scheduled
- Comfortable positions planned

Who touches first matters:

- More anxious partner often receives first
- 15-20 minutes each turn
- Clear transition between roles
- No simultaneous touching initially
- Receiver's only job: notice sensations

The toucher explores with curiosity:

- How does this texture feel to my fingers?
- What's the temperature difference here?
- How does pressure change the experience?
- What patterns feel interesting to create?

Touch techniques expand beyond basic rubbing:

Temperature play:

- Warm hands before starting
- Cool washcloth on warm skin
- Breath creating temperature shifts
- Ice cube traced lightly (advanced)

Pressure variations:

- Feather-light trailing
- Firm palm pressure
- Fingernail scratching
- Knuckle kneading
- Full hand holding

Texture exploration:

- Silk scarf dragging
- Fur or fleece brushing
- Your hair as a brush
- Different fabrics
- Lotion versus oil versus powder

Staying present when your mind wanders (and it will):

Notice the departure: "Oh, I'm thinking about work" No judgment: "Of course my mind wandered, that's normal" Gentle return: Focus on one specific sensation Anchor points: Temperature, texture, pressure, movement Breathe consciously: Links you to body

The receiver practices pure receiving:

- No reciprocating
- No performing pleasure
- No guiding or directing (initially)
- Just notice and breathe

- Mental notes of what feels good

Communication without words prevents performance pressure from sneaking back in. Talking about what feels good sounds helpful but often creates subtle demands.

Hand-riding technique:

- Receiver places hand over toucher's hand
- Guides pressure and movement silently
- Teaches preferences without words
- Toucher learns through feeling
- Creates intuitive understanding

Non-verbal sounds allowed:

- Sighs of pleasure
- Breathing changes
- Soft moans
- Not performed, just natural
- Toucher notices without pressure

Stage 2 adds face, neck, feet:

- More vulnerable areas
- Often surprisingly erotic
- Scalp massage discoveries
- Foot touching intimacy
- Face requires extra gentleness

Michael described his first session: "I kept waiting for it to get sexual. Then I realized my entire back was tingling, I was rock hard, and we hadn't gone near my penis. My wife was just trailing her fingers along my spine. I almost cried from how good it felt to just receive."

Stage 3-4: Including Erogenous Zones

Now things get interesting. You've spent weeks discovering pleasure without genital involvement. Your body has learned to relax, receive, and respond without pressure. Time to include the areas you've been avoiding—but with the same exploratory, non-goal approach.

Adding lubrication changes the entire sensory experience:

Choose quality lubricant:

- Silicone-based for longevity
- Water-based for easy cleanup
- Avoid numbing agents
- Fragrance-free preferred
- Warm in hands first

Lubrication everywhere:

- Not just genitals
- Inner thighs
- Lower belly
- Breasts/chest
- Anywhere skin touches skin

The sensation focus:

- How does slippery feel different?
- Temperature changes with moisture
- Pressure slides instead of drags
- New movements become possible

Genital touch without goals requires mental discipline:

For the toucher:

- Explore like unknown territory
- Notice textures, temperatures

73

- No technique, just curiosity
- Avoid stimulation patterns
- Think discovery, not arousal

For the receiver:

- Arousal is okay but not the point
- Notice without chasing sensation
- Erections may come and go
- No performing response
- Just breathe and feel

Common reactions:

- Anxiety about arousal level
- Frustration with exploration pace
- Desire to shift to "real" sex
- Performance thoughts returning
- Body responding differently

Managing arousal becomes the real practice:

When arousal builds:

- Notice without attachment
- Breathe deeply
- Shift touch to less sensitive areas
- Return when intensity decreases
- Practice arousal tolerance

The wave principle:

- Arousal naturally ebbs and flows
- Stop fighting the rhythm
- Ride waves without forcing
- Trust your body's wisdom
- Each wave teaches something

Mutual touching introduction in Stage 4:

Start position matters:

- Side by side
- Heads at opposite ends
- Can see but not faces
- Reduces performance pressure

Guidelines:

- Still no goals
- Focus on own sensation
- Not trying to arouse partner
- Notice giving and receiving
- Stop if overwhelming

Advanced variations:

- Sitting facing each other
- One active, one still
- Trading every few minutes
- Eye contact if comfortable
- Building to simultaneous

Sarah shared her breakthrough: "For twenty years, touching my husband's penis meant trying to make him come. During sensate focus, I just explored—the different textures, how it changed with touch, the warmth. He said it was the most erotic experience we'd had in years, and I never once tried to arouse him."

Stage 5: Sensual Intercourse

Here's where most couples screw up everything they've built. They think "finally, real sex!" and abandon everything they've learned. Wrong. Stage 5 takes the same mindful, exploratory

approach and applies it to intercourse. This isn't the finish line—
it's another playground.

Mindful penetration flips the script on intercourse:

Initial position:

- Woman on top usually easier
- Allows her control of pace
- Man stays relatively still
- Focus on sensation, not thrusting

The insertion meditation:

- Pause at entrance
- Notice warmth, pressure
- Millimeter by millimeter entry
- Stop frequently
- Full presence with sensation

No thrusting initially:

- Just be connected
- Feel pulse, warmth, wetness
- Notice micro-movements
- Breathe together
- Stay for minutes

The insert-and-remove technique builds new neural pathways:

The practice:

1. Insert partially or fully
2. Pause and feel
3. Slowly withdraw completely
4. Pause and notice absence
5. Repeat multiple times

What this teaches:

- Penetration isn't about friction
- Connection exists in stillness
- Absence enhances presence
- Control over arousal
- Pleasure in the journey

Common challenges:

- Urge to thrust
- Erection fluctuations
- Female arousal changes
- Impatience with pace
- Old patterns returning

Breathing coordination deepens connection:

Synchronous breathing:

- Match inhales and exhales
- Creates energetic circuit
- Slows racing thoughts
- Builds intimacy
- Prevents quick finish

Opposite breathing:

- One inhales while other exhales
- Creates push-pull dynamic
- Can increase arousal
- Requires more attention
- Advanced practice

Breath and movement:

- Inhale on entry

- Exhale on withdrawal
- Pause between breaths
- Let breath guide pace
- Natural rhythm emerges

Expanding definitions beyond thrusting:

Circular movements:

- Hips rotate without thrusting
- Different angles stimulated
- Slower arousal build
- More female stimulation
- Sustainable longer

Pressure variations:

- Deep and still
- Shallow and moving
- Angles changing pressure
- Using furniture/pillows
- Finding sweet spots

Position experimentation:

- Not for variety's sake
- Each offers different sensations
- Some reduce stimulation
- Others increase connection
- Mindful transition between

Time distortion:

- Five minutes feels like forever
- Or hour passes instantly
- Presence alters perception
- No clock watching

- Duration becomes irrelevant

David's revelation: "We spent 40 minutes with me inside her, barely moving. Sometimes I'd soften, we'd wait, I'd harden again. No panic, no performance thoughts. Just... connection. When we finally allowed more movement, the orgasms were secondary to the intimacy we'd built."

Key Takeaways

Sensate focus succeeds by removing the very thing everyone chases—sexual outcomes. This paradox frees your body to respond naturally, without the crushing weight of performance expectations. Masters and Johnson's genius wasn't in discovering new techniques but in recognizing that goal-oriented sex creates the problems it's trying to solve.

Starting with non-genital touch rewires associations. Your skin becomes a playground again, not a testing ground. Pleasure exists everywhere, not just between your legs. When sexual touch finally returns, it carries new meaning—exploration instead of expectation.

Including erogenous zones without goals requires discipline most couples lack. The temptation to fall into old patterns— stimulation, arousal, orgasm—feels overwhelming. But staying present with sensation, allowing arousal without chasing it, builds capacities that transform your entire sexual experience.

Mindful intercourse isn't slow sex or tantric marathon sessions. It's presence over performance, sensation over stimulation, connection over conquest. The techniques—insert and remove, breathing coordination, minimal movement—teach your body new ways of experiencing pleasure.

The real transformation happens between your ears. When sex stops being pass/fail and becomes play, everything changes.

Performance anxiety has no ground to stand on when there's no performance to judge. Erectile dysfunction becomes irrelevant when erections aren't required. Premature ejaculation disappears when lasting longer isn't the goal.

Your body already knows how to experience pleasure. Sensate focus just removes the mental blocks preventing that natural response. Stop trying so hard. Start feeling instead.

Chapter 8: Advanced Techniques for Lasting Longer

Premature ejaculation is the sexual equivalent of a sneeze. You feel it building, try to stop it, and then... too late. Except unlike sneezing, this particular loss of control can devastate your confidence, strain your relationship, and turn sex from pleasure into panic. But here's what nobody tells you: lasting longer is a skill, not a gift. And like any skill, it can be learned.

The porn-fueled fantasy of pounding away for 45 minutes straight? Pure fiction that's screwing up real men's expectations. The average guy lasts 5-7 minutes during intercourse. That's normal. That's plenty. But if you're finishing in 30 seconds when you want 5 minutes, or 2 minutes when you want 10, these techniques will change your life. No numbing sprays, no thinking about baseball, just real control built through understanding and practice.

Understanding Ejaculation Control

Control starts with awareness. Most men have no idea what's actually happening in their bodies during arousal. They go from zero to explosion with no understanding of the stages in between. It's like trying to drive a car while blindfolded—of course you're going to crash.

The arousal scale from 1-10 provides your roadmap:

1-3: Initial interest and arousal

- Light tingling sensation
- Beginning of erection

- Relaxed breathing
- Easy to stop or redirect

4-6: Building excitement

- Full erection achieved
- Increased heart rate
- Heightened sensitivity
- Still have control options

7-8: High arousal zone

- Intense pleasure sensations
- Breathing becomes shallow
- Muscle tension increases
- Control becomes challenging

9: The warning zone

- Feeling of inevitability approaching
- Internal muscles beginning to contract
- Last chance for intervention
- Seconds from point of no return

10: Point of no return and ejaculation

- Ejaculatory inevitability
- No stopping possible
- Muscle contractions begin
- Game over (for now)

Point of no return deserves special attention. This is the ejaculatory inevitability—the moment when ejaculation becomes unstoppable even if all stimulation ceases. Learning to recognize your point of no return is like learning to brake before the cliff, not at the edge (Althof, 2014).

Physical signals include:

- Testicles drawing up tight
- Feeling of fullness at penis base
- Involuntary muscle contractions starting
- Warmth spreading from pelvis
- That "oh shit" moment of recognition

Sympathetic vs parasympathetic nervous system management makes or breaks control:

Sympathetic (fight or flight) = quick ejaculation:

- Activated by performance anxiety
- Shallow, rapid breathing
- Muscle tension throughout body
- Racing thoughts
- Body wants to finish fast and escape

Parasympathetic (rest and digest) = lasting power:

- Activated by relaxation
- Deep, slow breathing
- Relaxed muscles
- Present-moment awareness
- Body can sustain arousal

The cruel irony? Worrying about coming too fast activates the very system that makes you come fast. It's like quicksand—the harder you fight, the faster you sink.

Individual variation explains why your buddy's technique might not work for you:

Sensitivity levels vary:

- Glans (head) sensitivity differs drastically

- Frenulum responsiveness unique to each man
- Shaft sensitivity patterns individual
- What overwhelms one man barely registers for another

Arousal patterns differ:

- Some men climb steadily
- Others spike quickly then plateau
- Some have multiple peaks
- Learn your unique pattern

Recovery times vary:

- Refractory period from minutes to hours
- Age affects but doesn't determine
- Health status impacts significantly
- Second round often provides better control

Jake came to me frustrated: "I tried everything my friends suggested. Nothing works." We discovered his arousal pattern was unusual—he'd spike to 8 immediately, then hover there. Standard techniques assumed gradual building. Once we adapted techniques to his pattern, control improved dramatically.

Physical Control Methods

Your body already knows how to delay ejaculation. You do it every time you edge during masturbation, stopping just before climax. These techniques simply formalize and enhance what you instinctively discovered as a teenager. The difference? Now you'll do it with purpose and precision.

Stop-start technique delivers the most bang for your buck (pun intended). Research shows men using this method increase their intravaginal ejaculation latency time by an average of 7-9 minutes (Ventus et al., 2020).

Solo training protocol:

1. Stimulate to arousal level 7
2. Stop completely, hands off
3. Breathe deeply, relax muscles
4. Wait until arousal drops to 4-5
5. Resume stimulation
6. Repeat 3-4 cycles before allowing climax

Progressive difficulty:

- Week 1-2: Dry hand
- Week 3-4: Lubrication added
- Week 5-6: Vary speed and pressure
- Week 7-8: Add fantasy/visual stimulation
- Week 9+: Partner involvement

Partner application:

- Clear communication essential
- Partner stops when signaled
- No shame or frustration
- Resume when ready
- Celebrate small improvements

Squeeze method provides emergency braking when stop-start isn't enough:

The technique:

1. At arousal level 8-9
2. Thumb on frenulum (underside)
3. Two fingers on opposite side
4. Firm pressure 10-20 seconds
5. Reduces erection and arousal
6. Wait 30 seconds before resuming

Pressure points:

- Just below glans most effective
- Base squeeze for variation
- Partner can apply from any angle
- Pressure firm but not painful
- Works even during intercourse

Common mistakes:

- Squeezing too late
- Insufficient pressure
- Holding too long
- Using during ejaculation (pointless)
- Not communicating with partner

Edging practice builds control like weight training builds muscle:

Solo edging workout:

- 20-minute minimum sessions
- Reach level 8 at least 6 times
- Never exceed level 9
- Vary stimulation types
- Track progress weekly

Advanced edging:

- Multiple peaks within each level
- Hovering at specific levels
- Rapid ascent/descent practice
- Different positions
- Environmental distractions

The plateau method:

- Reach level 7
- Maintain for 5 minutes
- Neither increasing nor decreasing
- Requires exquisite control
- Builds staying power

Position strategies can add or subtract minutes:

Lasting longer positions:

- Woman on top (you relax)
- Side by side (less thrusting)
- Spooning (controlled depth)
- Standing (blood flow different)
- Edge of bed variations

Quick finish positions (avoid initially):

- Missionary (full control/pressure)
- Doggy style (deep penetration)
- Legs on shoulders (intense angle)
- Any position you fantasize about

Angle adjustments:

- Upward curve? Avoid positions hitting front wall
- Downward curve? Skip positions stimulating bottom
- Leftward/rightward curve? Adjust accordingly
- Straight? Lucky you, experiment freely

Mark practiced edging religiously for six weeks. "At first I could barely reach level 7 without losing it. Now I can hover at 8.5 for ten minutes. My wife thinks I'm a different man. Hell, I feel like a different man."

Mental Control Strategies

Your mind controls ejaculation more than your penis does. That's not new-age nonsense—it's neuroscience. The same brain that creates performance anxiety can create calm control. Mental techniques work because they change your nervous system state, not because they distract you from pleasure.

Arousal surfing treats excitement like waves in the ocean:

The surfing mindset:

- Waves will come (arousal builds)
- You can't stop waves (natural process)
- You can choose which to ride
- You can paddle away from big ones
- Wipeouts happen (accept, don't judge)

Practical application:

- Feel arousal building (wave approaching)
- Choose to ride or retreat
- Use breath to modulate intensity
- Stay present with sensation
- No fighting, just flowing

The key insight: Fighting arousal creates tension that accelerates ejaculation. Surfing arousal accepts and works with your body's rhythms.

Distraction vs presence represents the old way versus the new:

Old school distraction:

- Think about baseball/work/taxes
- Mentally disconnect from experience
- Reduces pleasure for everyone
- Creates performance anxiety
- Temporary fix at best

New school presence:

- Focus intently on specific sensations
- Her breathing, skin temperature, sounds
- Your hand on her hip
- The sheet texture under you
- Anything except your penis

Why presence works better:

- Keeps you in parasympathetic mode
- Maintains connection with partner
- Reduces spectatoring
- Pleasure without pressure
- Sustainable long-term

Breathing patterns directly control arousal:

The 4-6 breath:

- Inhale 4 counts through nose
- Exhale 6 counts through mouth
- Longer exhale activates parasympathetic
- Practice during non-sexual times
- Becomes automatic under pressure

Belly breathing:

- Hand on stomach
- Expand belly on inhale
- Contract on exhale
- Opposite of stress breathing
- Sends calm signals throughout body

Partner breathing:

- Match her rhythm

- Creates energetic connection
- Slows you both down
- Builds intimacy
- Natural pace control

Visualization techniques pre-program success:

Pre-sex visualization:

- See yourself in control
- Imagine using techniques successfully
- Feel the confidence
- Include partner's pleasure
- End with mutual satisfaction

During-sex imagery:

- Visualize arousal as color/temperature
- See it spreading slowly
- Imagine cooling/dimming at will
- Picture energy circulating, not building
- Create mental gauges and controls

The roots technique:

- Imagine roots growing from base of spine
- Deep into the earth
- Grounding excess energy
- Staying centered
- Particularly effective for anxious types

Carlos struggled with racing thoughts during sex. "My mind was like a hamster on speed." We developed his personal visualization: seeing arousal as water filling a series of pools, each overflowing slowly to the next. "Now I can mentally control which pool fills. Sounds weird, but it works."

Partner Collaboration

Lasting longer isn't a solo sport. Your partner holds half the keys to your success. Yet most couples never discuss pace, pressure, or preferences. They fumble through sex hoping things magically improve. Spoiler alert: they don't. Clear communication and collaboration transform frustrating quickies into satisfying sessions.

Communication during sex requires overcoming the myth that good lovers read minds:

Verbal cues that work:

- "Let's slow down"
- "I need a break"
- "Let's switch"
- "Just like that"
- "Don't stop" (when sustainable)

Creating code words:

- "Yellow" = slow down
- "Red" = stop immediately
- "Green" = keep going
- Whatever feels natural
- Practice during low-pressure times

Non-verbal communication:

- Hand on hip to guide pace
- Gentle pressure to slow
- Pulling closer to deepen
- Breathing changes as signals
- Agreed-upon touches

Partner's verbal support:

- "We have all night"
- "I love feeling you inside me"
- "Take your time"
- "This feels amazing"
- Never "Are you close?" (pressure)

Pace control agreements establish who leads when:

The conversation starter: "I'd like to last longer for both of us. Can we work together on pacing?"

Options to discuss:

- She controls pace initially
- Switch leadership mid-session
- Verbal check-ins every few minutes
- Safe words for pace changes
- Celebration of small wins

Common rhythms:

- Start slow, build gradually
- Waves of intensity
- Plateau periods
- Position changes as breaks
- Her orgasm first, pressure off

Switching activities builds variety while providing breaks:

Natural transition points:

- Every 3-5 minutes initially
- When approaching level 7
- After position changes
- Between her orgasms
- Whenever either needs

Activity options:

- Oral (giving focuses outside yourself)
- Manual stimulation
- Kissing and caressing
- Toy involvement
- Sensual massage
- Dirty talk

The key: These aren't "breaks" from "real sex." They're part of the full experience. Remove the hierarchy that penetration matters most.

Aftercare importance often gets overlooked:

Regardless of duration:

- Cuddle and connect
- Express appreciation
- Avoid apologizing for timing
- Focus on what worked
- Plan improvements together

Processing together:

- "What felt best?"
- "What should we try next time?"
- "I loved when you..."
- No performance reviews
- Build positive associations

Building on success:

- Celebrate 30-second improvements
- Notice pattern changes
- Acknowledge effort
- Plan next experiments

- Keep it playful

Rachel and Tom transformed their sex life through collaboration: "We used to avoid talking during sex. Now we're constantly communicating—words, touches, sounds. Last night we made love for 45 minutes, switching between activities. Two months ago, Tom lasted 90 seconds. The difference? We're truly working together."

Key Takeaways

Ejaculation control is exactly that—control, not suppression. Understanding your arousal scale from 1-10 gives you a map of your body's responses. Recognizing point of no return means knowing when to brake. Managing your nervous system determines your staying power more than any technique.

Physical methods work because they formalize what your body already knows. Stop-start technique builds control systematically. The squeeze provides emergency braking. Edging practice develops mastery through repetition. Position strategies use physics to your advantage.

Mental control often matters more than physical. Arousal surfing replaces fighting with flowing. Presence beats distraction every time. Breathing patterns directly influence your nervous system. Visualization pre-programs success.

Partner collaboration multiplies your effectiveness. Communication during sex removes guesswork. Pace control agreements establish workable rhythms. Switching activities provides natural breaks without breaking connection. Aftercare builds positive associations regardless of duration.

The goal isn't porn-star stamina—it's mutual satisfaction. Most women don't want marathon sessions. They want present,

connected partners who last long enough for mutual pleasure.
That might be 5 minutes or 50, but it's definitely not 5 seconds.

Control is learnable. Practice builds competence.
Communication enables collaboration. Together, they transform
premature ejaculation from shameful secret to solved problem.

Your timing doesn't define you. But with these techniques, you
can define your timing.

Chapter 9: Age-Specific Strategies and Adaptations

Your penis doesn't come with an expiration date. But listening to most men talk, you'd think sexual function drops dead at 40, gets buried at 50, and haunts you as a ghost at 60. Complete nonsense. Sexual health changes with age, sure. But change doesn't mean decline—it means adaptation. And men who adapt thrive sexually into their 80s and beyond.

The real problem? We're using 20-year-old strategies for 50-year-old bodies. That's like wearing your high school letterman jacket to a business meeting—it doesn't fit, looks ridiculous, and everyone knows you're stuck in the past. Each decade brings unique challenges and opportunities. Understanding and working with these changes, instead of fighting them, transforms aging from sexual death sentence to natural evolution.

In Your 20s-30s: Prevention and Foundation

Young men think they're invincible. Morning erections like clockwork, recovery time measured in minutes, sexual thoughts every 7 seconds (that stat's bogus, by the way). Then suddenly, that first failure hits. Maybe after a night of heavy drinking. Maybe during a stressful period. And panic sets in because nobody prepared you for normal variations.

Addressing performance anxiety dominates this age group. Studies show 8-11% of men in their 20s now experience ED, compared to less than 2% just 20 years ago (Rastrelli & Maggi, 2017). What changed? Not biology—psychology.

Modern pressures creating anxiety:

- Porn setting impossible standards
- Hook-up culture performance pressure
- Social media comparison culture
- Dating app disposability mindset
- Work stress starting earlier
- Student debt crushing confidence

The anxiety spiral starts young:

1. One "failure" during stressed period
2. Worry about it happening again
3. Anxiety during next encounter
4. Self-fulfilling prophecy
5. Avoidance of intimacy
6. Identity crisis ("Am I broken?")

Breaking the spiral early:

- Normalize occasional difficulties
- Understand stress impacts
- Learn anxiety management now
- Build communication skills
- Develop body awareness
- Create healthy patterns

Building healthy habits early sets the foundation for decades:

Exercise habits to establish:

- 150 minutes cardio weekly minimum
- 2-3 strength training sessions
- Daily movement practice
- Flexibility/mobility work
- Sports for fun, not just fitness
- Partner activities when possible

Nutritional foundations:

- Learn to cook real food
- Limit processed crap now
- Moderate alcohol consumption
- Stay hydrated consistently
- Experiment with what energizes you
- Don't diet, create sustainable patterns

Sleep non-negotiables:

- 7-9 hours consistently
- Same bedtime/wake time
- Bedroom for sleep and sex only
- No screens in bed
- Learn your optimal temperature
- Invest in quality mattress

Managing porn influence requires honest conversation:

The porn problem:

- Average first exposure: age 11-13
- Creates unrealistic expectations
- Promotes performance over pleasure
- Reduces partner satisfaction
- Can create dependency
- Interferes with real intimacy

Reality checks needed:

- Average erection: 5.1 inches (not 8+)
- Average intercourse: 5-7 minutes (not 45)
- Most women don't orgasm from penetration
- Real sex includes awkwardness
- Bodies make weird sounds
- Nobody looks airbrushed during sex

Healthy relationship with porn:

- Limit frequency and duration
- Choose ethical, realistic content
- Never during relationship conflicts
- Discuss boundaries with partner
- Take regular breaks
- Notice impact on real sex

Relationship skills development matters more than penis size:

Communication patterns to build:

- Express needs without demanding
- Listen without defending
- Share vulnerabilities safely
- Negotiate differences respectfully
- Appreciate daily
- Fight fairly

Sexual communication specifically:

- Likes and dislikes
- Fantasies and boundaries
- Health concerns openly
- Performance pressures
- Satisfaction beyond orgasm
- Growth mindset about sex

Kevin, 26, came in panicked after two ED episodes. "I'm broken. This shouldn't happen at my age." We discovered he was working 70-hour weeks, drinking heavily to "relax," sleeping 4 hours nightly, and comparing himself to porn. Not broken—overwhelmed. Six weeks of lifestyle changes and anxiety management: "I feel like myself again. Actually, better than before."

In Your 40s: The Transition Years

Welcome to the decade where shit gets real. Your metabolism slows, responsibilities multiply, and that invincible feeling becomes a distant memory. But here's the secret: your 40s can be your sexual prime if you stop trying to be 25 and start optimizing for who you are now.

Early intervention importance cannot be overstated. This is when small problems become big ones if ignored:

Warning signs to address immediately:

- Morning erections less frequent
- Longer recovery between sessions
- Decreased spontaneous desire
- Softer erections
- Energy drops
- Weight gain around middle
- Sleep quality declining

Why intervention matters now:

- Easier to prevent than reverse
- Habits still changeable
- Partners more understanding
- Time to experiment
- Resources available
- Motivation high

The "wait and see" trap:

- Problems rarely improve alone
- Shame builds with time
- Partner resentment grows
- Physical issues compound
- Confidence erodes
- Options narrow

Hormone optimization naturally becomes crucial:

Testosterone facts for 40s:

- Drops 1-2% yearly after 30
- Stress accelerates decline
- Belly fat converts T to estrogen
- Sleep deprivation crashes levels
- Most men still in normal range
- Optimization different from replacement

Natural optimization strategies:

- Heavy compound lifts 2x weekly
- HIIT training for hormone spike
- Vitamin D3 optimization
- Zinc and magnesium supplementation
- Stress reduction priority
- 7-9 hours sleep non-negotiable

Diet for hormones:

- Healthy fats 30% of calories
- Cruciferous vegetables daily
- Limited sugar and processed foods
- Moderate alcohol only
- Intermittent fasting benefits
- Cholesterol isn't enemy

Stress management priorities shift in your 40s:

Common stressors peaking:

- Career pressures/plateau
- Teenage children
- Aging parents
- Financial pressures

- Relationship staleness
- Physical changes
- Existential questions

Stress impacts everything:

- Cortisol suppresses testosterone
- Kills spontaneous desire
- Disrupts sleep
- Increases belly fat
- Raises blood pressure
- Clouds mental clarity

Effective management for busy 40s:

- Morning meditation 10 minutes
- Walking meetings when possible
- Saying no to non-essentials
- Date nights scheduled
- Solo time protected
- Hobbies maintained

Preventive cardiovascular care protects future function:

Your erection is your check engine light:

- ED often precedes heart disease by 3-5 years
- Same vessels, same problems
- Prevention now saves function later
- Partners motivate better health
- Sex improves with cardiovascular fitness

Key metrics to monitor:

- Blood pressure under 120/80
- LDL cholesterol under 100
- Triglycerides under 150

- Fasting glucose under 100
- Waist under 40 inches
- Resting heart rate under 70

Action steps:

- Annual physical with full labs
- Cardiovascular exercise priority
- Mediterranean diet adoption
- Stress reduction techniques
- Weight management
- Partner involvement

Marcus, 45, ignored subtle changes for three years. "I figured it was normal aging." By the time he sought help, he had full ED, prediabetes, and hypertension. Took 18 months to reverse. His brother, 43, saw Marcus's struggle and addressed early symptoms immediately. Six months of intervention: "I feel better than I did at 35."

In Your 50s-60s: Adaptation and Optimization

This is where boys become men and men become wise. Your body changes more noticeably, but your experience, confidence, and emotional intelligence peak. The men who thrive sexually in this decade are those who adapt gracefully rather than desperately clinging to youth.

Working with physical changes requires acceptance plus action:

Normal changes to expect:

- Erections take longer to achieve
- May need direct stimulation

- Less rigid when standing
- Longer refractory period
- Decreased spontaneous erections
- Lower ejaculate volume
- Orgasm intensity varies

What's NOT normal:

- Complete inability to achieve erection
- Pain during arousal or orgasm
- Significant size changes
- Curved erection (new onset)
- Blood in semen
- Urination difficulties

Adaptation strategies:

- Allow more warm-up time
- Use lubricant liberally
- Try cock rings for maintenance
- Explore different positions
- Focus on whole-body pleasure
- Communicate needs openly

Medical condition management becomes central:

Common conditions affecting function:

- Type 2 diabetes (damages vessels/nerves)
- Hypertension (medication side effects)
- Heart disease (circulation issues)
- Prostate enlargement (urinary/sexual)
- Arthritis (position limitations)
- Depression (desire and function)

Medication considerations:

- Many BP meds affect erections
- Antidepressants delay orgasm
- Statins may impact testosterone
- Prostate meds alter ejaculation
- Always discuss sexual side effects
- Often alternatives available

Working with your doctor:

- Be honest about sexual health
- Bring partner to appointments
- Ask about medication alternatives
- Discuss all supplements
- Request hormone testing
- Don't accept "just age"

Testosterone considerations get complex:

Natural strategies first:

- Resistance training crucial
- Weight loss if needed
- Sleep optimization
- Stress management
- Nutritional support
- Limit alcohol

Testing considerations:

- Total and free testosterone
- Multiple morning samples
- Consider symptoms, not just numbers
- SHBG affects availability
- Estradiol balance matters
- Full hormone panel

Replacement therapy questions:

- Benefits vs risks individual
- Multiple delivery methods
- Requires ongoing monitoring
- Not a magic bullet
- Partner involvement important
- Lifestyle still matters

Intimacy evolution creates new possibilities:

Expanding definitions:

- Sensual massage importance
- Oral sex excellence
- Manual techniques mastery
- Toy integration
- Fantasy exploration
- Emotional intimacy deepening

Quality over quantity shift:

- Weekly vs daily perfectly normal
- Longer, more intentional sessions
- Planning enhances anticipation
- Morning often better
- Vacation sex renaissance
- Connection over performance

Partner considerations:

- Menopause affects her too
- Lubricant essential
- More foreplay needed
- Communication crucial
- Health issues mutual
- Growing together

William, 58, embraced changes: "I stopped trying to fuck like a 30-year-old and started making love like a 58-year-old. Game changer. We have the best sex of our marriage. Less frequent, but more connected. My wife says I'm finally present instead of performing."

70s and Beyond: Intimacy Without Limits

Society desexualizes older adults like they're Ken dolls—smooth plastic where genitals should be. Bullshit. Research shows people remain sexual beings until death. The expression changes, but the desire for connection, pleasure, and intimacy continues. Men in their 70s, 80s, and beyond can have deeply satisfying sexual lives—they just need to redefine what that means.

Redefining sexual expression opens new worlds:

Broader definition includes:

- Naked cuddling
- Sensual bathing together
- Full-body massage
- Kissing sessions
- Manual pleasuring
- Oral exploration
- Mutual masturbation
- Fantasy sharing

Pleasure without pressure:

- Erections appreciated, not required
- Orgasm optional
- Duration irrelevant
- Connection paramount

- Creativity encouraged
- Laughter welcomed

Morning intimacy advantages:

- Testosterone highest
- Energy levels better
- Less distraction
- Natural light
- Relaxed pace
- Sets positive day tone

Medication interactions require careful management:

Common medications affecting function:

- Heart medications (most)
- Diabetes medications
- Antidepressants
- Pain medications
- Prostate medications
- Parkinson's drugs

Safety considerations:

- Nitrates and ED drugs don't mix
- Blood pressure monitoring
- Heart condition clearance
- Stroke risk assessment
- Balance issues with positions
- Hydration importance

Working with multiple doctors:

- Keep all informed
- Bring medication list
- Partner advocates help

- Pharmacist consultations
- Regular reviews
- Adjustment willingness

Partner health considerations become mutual:

Common partner issues:

- Vaginal dryness/atrophy
- Decreased libido
- Pain during intercourse
- Chronic health conditions
- Mobility limitations
- Body image concerns

Mutual adaptations:

- Simultaneous position adjustments
- Shared medical appointments
- Exercise together
- Nutritional changes mutual
- Sleep optimization
- Stress reduction partnership

Communication evolution:

- More direct about needs
- Less assumption
- Check-ins during activity
- Appreciation expressed
- Frustrations acknowledged
- Solutions collaborative

Quality over quantity becomes wisdom:

What matters most:

- Being desired
- Feeling connected
- Sharing pleasure
- Maintaining intimacy
- Creating joy
- Expressing love

Success redefined:

- "We touched lovingly"
- "We laughed together"
- "We felt close"
- "We gave pleasure"
- "We were present"
- "We connected"

George, 78, shared wisdom: "My erection works about half the time. Used to devastate me. Now? We've discovered fifty ways to pleasure each other. My hands work fine. My mouth works great. My heart works perfectly. We're having more fun in bed than we've had in decades. Just took changing my definition of sex."

Key Takeaways

Sexual health isn't static—it evolves throughout life. Each decade brings unique challenges and opportunities. Men who adapt thrive; those who resist suffer unnecessarily.

Your 20s and 30s are for building foundations. Address performance anxiety early. Create healthy habits now that serve you forever. Manage porn's influence. Develop relationship skills that matter more than penis size.

Your 40s demand attention and intention. Early intervention prevents major problems. Natural hormone optimization works if you work it. Stress management becomes non-negotiable. Cardiovascular health determines sexual future.

Your 50s and 60s reward adaptation. Physical changes are normal, not catastrophic. Medical condition management requires partnership with healthcare. Testosterone needs individual consideration. Intimacy evolution creates new possibilities.

Your 70s and beyond offer unlimited intimacy potential. Redefining sexual expression opens new pleasures. Medication interactions need careful management. Partner health considerations become mutual adventures. Quality trumps quantity every time.

The thread connecting every decade? Men who stay curious, communicative, and creative maintain satisfying sexual lives regardless of age. Your penis might change, but your capacity for pleasure, connection, and intimacy only grows—if you let it.

Age is just a number. Adaptation is everything.

Chapter 10: Creating Your Personalized Action Plan

Knowledge without action is like having a map but never leaving your driveway. You've learned about the mind-body connection, exercise protocols, nutrition strategies, sleep optimization, communication techniques, and age-specific adaptations. Great. Now what? This chapter transforms all that information into your personal roadmap for sexual health transformation.

Here's the thing most self-help books won't tell you: reading doesn't change anything. Action does. But not random action—strategic, progressive, personalized action that builds momentum while respecting your unique situation. One size fits nobody. Your plan needs to fit your life, your relationship, your challenges, and your goals. So let's build it together.

Week 1-2: Foundation Building

Starting is the hardest part. Your brain will find a thousand reasons to wait until Monday, next month, after the holidays, when life calms down (spoiler: it never does). But sexual health doesn't improve through procrastination. It improves through small, consistent actions starting right now.

Initial assessment completion gives you a baseline to measure progress against. You can't know if you're improving without knowing where you started.

Take the IIEF-5 questionnaire (from Chapter 1):

- Rate your confidence in getting erections
- Assess hardness levels
- Evaluate maintenance ability

- Note satisfaction levels
- Calculate your total score
- Write it down with today's date

Additional baseline measurements:

- Morning erections per week
- Energy levels (1-10 scale)
- Stress levels (1-10 scale)
- Relationship satisfaction
- Current medications
- Sleep quality assessment

Physical markers to record:

- Weight and waist measurement
- Blood pressure if possible
- Resting heart rate
- Flexibility (touch toes?)
- How many flights of stairs wind you
- Current exercise frequency

Communication groundwork with your partner prevents misunderstandings and builds support:

The conversation starter: "I've been reading about men's sexual health, and I want to make some changes to improve things for both of us. Would you be open to supporting me in this?"

Topics to cover:

- Your goals (be specific)
- Changes they might notice
- How they can help
- Their concerns or goals
- Schedule for check-ins
- Celebration plans

If single, identify support:

- Trusted friend
- Online community
- Therapist
- Men's group
- Anyone who'll provide accountability

Basic Kegel routine starts immediately because it requires no equipment, no gym, no special time:

Week 1 protocol:

- Find the muscles (stop urination test)
- 10 quick contractions, 3x daily
- 5 three-second holds, 3x daily
- Do them everywhere (car, desk, couch)
- No breath holding
- No glute engagement

Common mistakes already:

- Overdoing it (muscles need recovery)
- Involving abs or glutes
- Forgetting to breathe
- Expecting instant results
- Doing them only lying down

Sleep optimization begins with assessment and simple changes:

Current sleep audit:

- Track bedtime/wake time for 3 nights
- Note how long to fall asleep
- Count night wakings
- Rate morning energy
- Identify sleep thieves

Immediate changes to implement:

- Set consistent bedtime (within 30 minutes)
- Phone charging outside bedroom
- Room temperature 65-68°F
- Blackout curtains or eye mask
- No screens 1 hour before bed
- Morning sunlight within 30 minutes of waking

Dietary cleanup starts with elimination, not addition:

Week 1-2 eliminations:

- Sugary drinks (all of them)
- Processed snacks from house
- Fast food meals
- Excess alcohol (max 2 drinks when drinking)
- Late-night eating (stop 3 hours before bed)

Don't try to overhaul everything. Just stop putting garbage in your body while you figure out what to add.

Michael started enthusiastically: "I'm going to exercise daily, meditate for an hour, completely change my diet, and do Kegels every hour!" He lasted three days. His second attempt: "I'll do 10 Kegels three times daily and stop drinking soda." Six months later, he'd built on that foundation to transform his entire lifestyle. Start small. Build steadily.

Week 3-4: Momentum Building

Two weeks in, the honeymoon phase ends. Initial enthusiasm wanes. Old habits whisper sweet temptations. This is where most men quit. But you're not most men. You've built a foundation. Now we add the next layer.

Exercise routine establishment can't wait any longer:

115

Minimum effective dose:

- 3x weekly 30-minute walks (or equivalent)
- 2x weekly basic strength training
- Daily 5-minute morning movement

Week 3 starter routine: Monday: 30-minute brisk walk Tuesday: Basic strength (push-ups, squats, planks) Wednesday: 30-minute walk Thursday: Rest or gentle yoga Friday: Basic strength session Weekend: One fun physical activity

Week 4 progression:

- Increase walk pace or duration
- Add 1-2 strength exercises
- Include hills or stairs
- Try one HIIT session
- Partner involvement if possible

Mindfulness practice daily doesn't mean becoming a monk:

10-minute starter practice:

- 2 minutes settling in
- 6 minutes breath awareness
- 2 minutes body scan
- That's it

Where to practice:

- First thing morning (before phone)
- Lunch break in car
- Before bed
- During commute (not driving)
- Bathroom breaks at work

Apps that actually help:

- Headspace (beginner-friendly)
- Calm (sleep stories bonus)
- Insight Timer (free options)
- Ten Percent Happier (skeptic-friendly)

The key: consistency over perfection. Two minutes daily beats 20 minutes once a week.

Sensate focus stage 1 begins the intimacy journey:

First session setup:

- 30-45 minutes scheduled
- Warm room, soft lighting
- No genital contact allowed
- One person touches, one receives
- 15-20 minutes each role
- No talking during

Focus areas for stage 1:

- Back exploration
- Arms and hands
- Legs and feet
- Neck and shoulders
- Face and scalp
- Notice temperature, texture, response

After-session discussion:

- What felt surprisingly good?
- Any anxiety or thoughts?
- Moments of presence?
- Want to adjust anything?

Nutritional enhancement adds NO-boosting foods:

Daily additions week 3:

- Morning: 8oz beet juice or 1 roasted beet
- Lunch: Large dark leafy salad
- Snack: 1oz dark chocolate (70%+)
- Dinner: Include garlic and olive oil

Week 4 additions:

- Watermelon juice (16oz) on workout days
- Handful of walnuts daily
- Pomegranate juice option
- Fatty fish 2x weekly

Keep eliminations from weeks 1-2 while adding these enhancers.

Stress reduction techniques become daily practice:

The 4-7-8 breath for acute stress:

- Inhale 4 counts
- Hold 7 counts
- Exhale 8 counts
- Repeat 4 cycles
- Use before any stressful event

Box breathing for meetings:

- In 4, hold 4, out 4, hold 4
- Can do invisibly
- Activates parasympathetic
- Improves focus too

Progressive muscle relaxation before bed:

- Start with toes

- Tense 5 seconds
- Release and notice
- Move up body
- Takes 10-15 minutes total

David reported at week 4: "I'm sleeping better, my energy's up, and morning erections are back some days. My wife says I seem calmer. We haven't even addressed the sexual stuff directly yet, but I already feel different."

Month 2-3: Integration and Advancement

Now you're cooking. The basics have become routine. Sleep is improving. Exercise feels normal. Stress is manageable. Time to level up everything while adding targeted interventions. This phase separates those who get temporary improvement from those who transform their lives.

Progressive exercise intensity builds on your foundation:

Month 2 cardio progression:

- Increase duration to 40 minutes
- Add interval training 1x weekly
- Include incline/resistance
- Track heart rate zones
- Swimming or cycling variety

Month 2 strength advancement:

- Add weight or resistance
- Include compound movements
- Focus on progressive overload
- Core work emphasis
- Recovery days sacred

Month 3 optimization:

- HIIT 2x weekly
- Strength training 3x weekly
- Active recovery days
- Flexibility work included
- Partner workouts when possible

Advanced Kegel variations target different muscle fibers:

Quick-twitch development:

- 1-second rapid contractions
- 30 reps
- Rest 30 seconds
- Repeat 3 sets
- 2x daily

Endurance holds:

- 10-second holds
- 10 reps
- Focus on consistent pressure
- No cheating with glutes
- Daily practice

Functional training:

- Kegels during squats
- Standing variations
- Different positions
- During partner activities
- Throughout daily life

Sensate focus progression moves through stages:

Month 2: Include stage 2-3

- Face and neck touching added
- Feet exploration
- Still no genital contact
- Building anticipation
- Deepening presence

Month 3: Progress to stage 4

- Genital touching allowed
- No orgasm goals
- Include lubrication
- Explore without agenda
- Communication evolving

Signs you're ready to progress:

- Comfortable with current stage
- Minimal performance thoughts
- Partner engaged and enjoying
- Presence increasing
- Anxiety decreasing

Supplement optimization adds targeted support:

Month 2 additions:

- Vitamin D3: 3000-5000 IU daily
- Zinc: 15-30mg daily
- Magnesium glycinate: 400mg before bed
- Omega-3: 2g EPA/DHA daily

Month 3 performance additions:

- L-citrulline: 1.5g daily
- Or L-arginine: 3-5g daily
- Ashwagandha: 600mg for stress
- B-complex for energy

Quality matters:

- Third-party tested brands
- Check expiration dates
- Store properly
- Track effects
- Adjust based on response

Relationship deepening through emotional intimacy exercises:

Daily appreciations:

- Share 3 things you appreciate
- Be specific
- Include non-physical qualities
- Write them sometimes
- Express genuinely

Weekly deep talks:

- 30 minutes uninterrupted
- Phones away
- Take turns sharing
- Dreams and fears included
- Physical touch while talking

Monthly adventures:

- New experiences together
- Doesn't require expense
- Build shared memories
- Laugh together
- Celebrate progress

Carlos at month 3: "I can't believe the change. I'm down 15 pounds, blood pressure normal, and we're having sex twice a week—good sex. My wife and I talk more in one week than we used to in a month. Kegels are automatic now. I actually look forward to exercise. Is this what healthy feels like?"

Long-term Sustainability

The real test isn't the first three months—it's month six, year two, decade later. Most men ride initial motivation to quick improvements, then slide back to old patterns. Sustainability requires systems, not willpower. Let's build yours.

3-month evaluation shows what's working:

Quantitative measurements:

- Retake IIEF-5, compare scores
- Morning erections per week
- Exercise sessions completed
- Weight and waist changes
- Blood pressure improvements
- Sleep quality scores

Qualitative assessments:

- Energy levels throughout day
- Stress management ability
- Relationship satisfaction
- Confidence changes
- Overall well-being
- Partner feedback

What to adjust:

- Exercises that bore you
- Unsustainable restrictions
- Supplements not helping
- Techniques not resonating
- Communication patterns

- Unrealistic expectations

6-month optimization fine-tunes everything:

Exercise evolution:

- Find activities you love
- Join groups or classes
- Set performance goals
- Try new modalities
- Make it social

Nutritional sustainability:

- 80/20 rule (good/flex)
- Meal prep strategies
- Restaurant navigation
- Travel planning
- Special occasion balance

Relationship momentum:

- Regular date nights
- Annual romantic getaways
- Continued sensate focus
- New experiences together
- Keep talking

Annual health checks monitor biomarkers:

Essential tests:

- Complete blood count
- Comprehensive metabolic panel
- Lipid panel
- Hormone panel (testosterone, thyroid)
- Vitamin D levels

- Inflammatory markers
- Prostate checks age-appropriate

Track trends, not single values:

- Direction matters more than number
- Annual comparisons
- Medication adjustments
- Supplement modifications
- Lifestyle correlations

Lifestyle integration makes healthy automatic:

Habit stacking mastery:

- Kegels with existing habits
- Exercise with commute
- Meditation with morning routine
- Supplements with meals
- Couple time scheduled

Environmental design:

- Workout clothes visible
- Healthy snacks accessible
- Bedroom optimized
- Supplements organized
- Barriers removed

Continuous learning keeps you engaged:

Stay informed through:

- Reputable health websites
- New research findings
- Community discussions
- Professional consultations

- Partner feedback
- Body awareness

But don't chase every fad:

- Stick with proven basics
- Test one change at a time
- Give changes 6-8 weeks
- Trust your experience
- Partner input matters

Troubleshooting Common Challenges

Real life doesn't follow neat chapters. You'll hit plateaus, face setbacks, encounter resistance, struggle with time, and question everything. That's not failure—that's the process. Here's how to navigate the inevitable obstacles.

Plateau breaking when progress stalls:

Why plateaus happen:

- Body adapts to stimulus
- Complacency sets in
- Stress increases elsewhere
- Hormones fluctuate
- Seasons change

Plateau-busting strategies:

- Change exercise completely for 2 weeks
- Try intermittent fasting
- Get hormone levels checked
- Take a full rest week
- Recommit to basics
- Seek professional guidance

The mental game:

- Plateaus are normal
- Not permanent
- Often precede breakthroughs
- Time to experiment
- Patience required

Setback management for temporary failures:

Common setbacks:

- Stress-induced ED return
- Old habits creeping back
- Injury disrupting exercise
- Relationship conflicts
- Health issues arising

Recovery protocol:

- Don't catastrophize
- Return to basics immediately
- Communicate with partner
- Adjust expectations temporarily
- Focus on what you can control
- Learn from the experience

The two-day rule:

- One day off is life
- Two days starts a pattern
- Never miss twice
- Applies to everything
- Builds resilience

Partner resistance navigation:

Why partners resist:

- Fear of change
- Their own insecurities
- Past disappointments
- Different priorities
- Communication failures

Working through it:

- Start with listening
- Acknowledge their feelings
- Find common ground
- Start smaller
- Include their goals
- Consider couples therapy

When to proceed alone:

- Safety issues
- Absolute refusal
- Your health priority
- Model positive change
- Door stays open

Time management for busy lives:

Time audit reality check:

- Track one typical day
- Find the waste
- TV/social media time
- Inefficient routines
- Saying yes too much

Efficiency strategies:

- Morning routine optimization
- Lunch break workouts
- Walking meetings
- Couple workouts
- Kids included activities
- Weekend meal prep

The truth about time:

- Everyone has same 24 hours
- Priorities determine usage
- Health enables everything else
- Small blocks add up
- Consistency over duration

Maintaining motivation when enthusiasm fades:

Reconnect with your why:

- Original pain points
- Future vision
- Partner's needs
- Health scare prevention
- Life quality desires

Motivation sustainers:

- Track small wins
- Celebrate milestones
- Share successes
- Join communities
- Set new goals
- Help others

The discipline bridge:

- Motivation starts

- Discipline continues
- Habits sustain
- Identity shifts
- Becomes who you are

Success Metrics and Tracking

What gets measured gets managed. But measuring the wrong things leads to frustration. Success in sexual health isn't just about erection hardness or lasting longer—it's about overall life enhancement.

Quantitative measures provide objective data:

Sexual function metrics:

- IIEF-5 scores monthly
- Morning erections weekly
- Successful encounters
- Duration improvements
- Recovery time changes

Health markers:

- Weight and body composition
- Blood pressure trends
- Resting heart rate
- Exercise performance
- Sleep quality scores

Behavioral tracking:

- Workouts completed
- Meditation minutes
- Kegel consistency
- Supplement adherence
- Stress management use

Qualitative assessments capture what matters:

Confidence indicators:

- Initiation comfort
- Performance anxiety levels
- Body image improvements
- Social confidence
- Overall self-esteem

Connection measures:

- Communication quality
- Emotional intimacy
- Non-sexual affection
- Shared activities
- Conflict resolution

Pleasure factors:

- Enjoyment levels
- Presence during sex
- Variety exploration
- Playfulness return
- Satisfaction beyond orgasm

Partner feedback integration provides crucial perspective:

Regular check-ins include:

- What's improving?
- What needs work?
- How can I support you?
- What do you need?
- Are we growing together?

Creating safe feedback:

- No defensive responses
- Appreciate honesty
- Act on reasonable requests
- Share your experience too
- Celebrate together

Health marker monitoring catches issues early:

Home monitoring:

- Blood pressure weekly
- Weight weekly (same day/time)
- Waist measurement monthly
- Heart rate variability
- Energy levels daily

Professional monitoring:

- Annual full panel
- Quarterly if issues
- Medication adjustments
- Specialist referrals
- Preventive care

Celebrating victories fuels continued progress:

What to celebrate:

- First morning erection return
- Anxiety-free encounter
- Partner compliment
- Health marker improvement
- New personal record
- Helping another man

How to celebrate:

- Share with supporter
- Journal the victory
- Reward appropriately
- Tell your partner
- Post in community
- Plan next goal

Resources and Support

No man is an island, especially when addressing sexual health. The right support multiplies your chances of success. The wrong support (or isolation) guarantees struggle.

Finding qualified professionals when you need help:

AASECT certified therapists:

- Specialized training
- Sex-positive approach
- Evidence-based methods
- Couple or individual
- Directory available online

Medical professionals:

- Urologist for physical issues
- Endocrinologist for hormones
- Cardiologist for vascular
- Primary care coordination
- Functional medicine option

Other professionals:

- Pelvic floor physical therapist
- Registered dietitian
- Personal trainer
- Massage therapist

- Acupuncturist

Online communities provide 24/7 support:

Valuable communities offer:

- Anonymity if needed
- Shared experiences
- Success stories
- Practical advice
- Accountability partners

Red flags to avoid:

- Miracle cure promises
- Expensive programs
- Shame-based approaches
- Unmoderated spaces
- Commercial focus only

Recommended apps for tracking and training:

Meditation/Mindfulness:

- Headspace
- Calm
- Insight Timer
- Ten Percent Happier

Exercise/Health:

- MyFitnessPal
- Strava
- Nike Training Club
- Fitbit/Apple Health

Sleep:

- Sleep Cycle
- Pillow
- AutoSleep

Relationship:

- Lasting
- Relish
- Love Nudge

Further reading for deep dives:

Books worth your time:

- "Come As You Are" - Emily Nagoski
- "The New Male Sexuality" - Bernie Zilbergeld
- "Mating in Captivity" - Esther Perel
- "Why Zebras Don't Get Ulcers" - Robert Sapolsky
- "The Body Keeps the Score" - Bessel van der Kolk

Emergency protocols for crisis situations:

Seek immediate help for:

- Chest pain during sex
- Painful erections lasting hours
- Blood in semen/urine
- Sudden complete ED
- Severe depression
- Suicidal thoughts

Remember: Asking for help shows strength, not weakness.

Your Journey Forward

You now have everything needed to transform your sexual health. Not through pills or quick fixes, but through systematic lifestyle changes that improve everything about your life. The journey requires commitment, patience, and self-compassion. Some days will be harder than others. Progress won't be linear. But if you trust the process and stay consistent, transformation is inevitable.

Start today. Not tomorrow. Not Monday. Now. Pick one thing—just one—and begin. Maybe it's 10 Kegels. Maybe it's a walk around the block. Maybe it's an honest conversation with your partner. Whatever it is, do it today.

Your future self will thank you. Your partner will thank you. Most importantly, you'll thank yourself for finally taking action instead of just reading about it.

The plan is here. The tools are yours. The only question left: Will you use them?

Your sexual health journey doesn't end with this book—it begins. Welcome to the first day of your transformation.

Reference

1. Althof, S. E. (2006). Prevalence, characteristics and implications of premature ejaculation/rapid ejaculation. Journal of Urology, 175(3), 842-848.
2. Althof, S. E., McMahon, C. G., Waldinger, M. D., Serefoglu, E. C., Shindel, A. W., Adaikan, P. G., ... & Torres, L. O. (2014). An update of the International Society of Sexual Medicine's guidelines for the diagnosis and treatment of premature ejaculation. Sexual Medicine, 2(2), 60-90.
3. Andersson, K. E. (2011). Mechanisms of penile erection and basis for pharmacological treatment of erectile dysfunction. Pharmacological Reviews, 63(4), 811-859.
4. Burnett, A. L., Nehra, A., Breau, R. H., Culkin, D. J., Faraday, M. M., Hakim, L. S., ... & Shindel, A. W. (2018). Erectile dysfunction: AUA guideline. Journal of Urology, 200(3), 633-641.
5. Goldstein, I. (2000). The mutually reinforcing triad of depressive symptoms, cardiovascular disease, and erectile dysfunction. American Journal of Cardiology, 86(2), 41-45.
6. McCabe, M., Sharlip, I., Lewis, R., Atalla, E., Balon, R., Fisher, A., ... & Segraves, R. (2016). Incidence and prevalence of sexual dysfunction in women and men: A consensus statement from the Fourth International Consultation on Sexual Medicine. Journal of Sexual Medicine, 13(2), 144-152.
7. Meston, C. M., Levin, R. J., Sipski, M. L., Hull, E. M., & Heiman, J. R. (2004). Women's orgasm. Annual Review of Sex Research, 15(1), 173-257.
8. Nguyen, H. M. T., Gabrielson, A. T., & Hellstrom, W. J. (2017). Erectile dysfunction in young men—A review of the prevalence and risk factors. Sexual Medicine Reviews, 5(4), 508-520.
9. Rosen, R. C., Cappelleri, J. C., Smith, M. D., Lipsky, J., & Peña, B. M. (1997). Development and evaluation of an

abridged, 5-item version of the International Index of Erectile Function (IIEF-5) as a diagnostic tool for erectile dysfunction. International Journal of Impotence Research, 11(6), 319-326.

10. Shamloul, R., & Ghanem, H. (2013). Erectile dysfunction. The Lancet, 381(9861), 153-165.

11. Traish, A. M. (2014). Adverse health effects of testosterone deficiency in men. Steroids, 88, 106-116.

12. Bancroft, J., & Janssen, E. (2000). The dual control model of male sexual response: A theoretical approach to centrally mediated erectile dysfunction. Neuroscience & Biobehavioral Reviews, 24(5), 571-579.

13. Cascio, C. N., O'Donnell, M. B., Tinney, F. J., Lieberman, M. D., Taylor, S. E., Strecher, V. J., & Falk, E. B. (2016). Self-affirmation activates brain systems associated with self-related processing and reward. Social Cognitive and Affective Neuroscience, 11(4), 621-629.

14. Lutz, A., Greischar, L. L., Rawlings, N. B., Ricard, M., & Davidson, R. J. (2004). Long-term meditators self-induce high-amplitude gamma synchrony during mental practice. Proceedings of the National Academy of Sciences, 101(46), 16369-16373.

15. McCabe, M. P., Sharlip, I. D., Atalla, E., Balon, R., Fisher, A. D., Laumann, E., ... & Segraves, R. T. (2016). Definitions of sexual dysfunctions in women and men: A consensus statement from the Fourth International Consultation on Sexual Medicine. Journal of Sexual Medicine, 13(2), 135-143.

16. Rosen, R. C., Miner, M. M., & Wincze, J. P. (2014). Erectile dysfunction: Integration of medical and psychological approaches. In Y. M. Binik & K. S. K. Hall (Eds.), Principles and practice of sex therapy (5th ed., pp. 61-85). Guilford Press.

17. Stephenson, K. R., & Kerth, J. (2017). Effects of mindfulness-based therapies for female sexual

dysfunction: A meta-analytic review. Journal of Sex Research, 54(7), 832-849.

18. Waldinger, M. D. (2005). Lifelong premature ejaculation: From authority-based to evidence-based medicine. BJU International, 96(2), 191-205.

19. Bacon, C. G., Mittleman, M. A., Kawachi, I., Giovannucci, E., Glasser, D. B., & Rimm, E. B. (2003). Sexual function in men older than 50 years of age: Results from the health professionals follow-up study. Annals of Internal Medicine, 139(3), 161-168.

20. Dorey, G., Speakman, M. J., Feneley, R. C., Swinkels, A., & Dunn, C. D. (2005). Pelvic floor exercises for erectile dysfunction. BJU International, 96(4), 595-597.

21. Khoo, J., Tian, H. H., Tan, B., Chew, K., Ng, C. S., Leong, D., ... & Chen, R. Y. (2013). Comparing effects of low-and high-volume moderate-intensity exercise on sexual function and testosterone in obese men. Journal of Sexual Medicine, 10(7), 1823-1832.

22. Kraemer, W. J., & Ratamess, N. A. (2005). Hormonal responses and adaptations to resistance exercise and training. Sports Medicine, 35(4), 339-361.

23. Silva, A. B., Sousa, N., Azevedo, L. F., & Martins, C. (2017). Physical activity and exercise for erectile dysfunction: Systematic review and meta-analysis. British Journal of Sports Medicine, 51(19), 1419-1424.

24. Stafford, R. E., Ashton-Miller, J. A., Constantinou, C., Coughlin, G., Lutton, N. J., & Hodges, P. W. (2016). Pattern of activation of pelvic floor muscles in men differs with verbal instructions. Neurourology and Urodynamics, 35(4), 457-463.

25. Chen, J., Wollman, Y., Chernichovsky, T., Iaina, A., Sofer, M., & Matzkin, H. (1999). Effect of oral administration of high-dose nitric oxide donor L-arginine in men with organic erectile dysfunction: Results of a double-blind, randomized, placebo-controlled study. BJU International, 83(3), 269-273.

26. Cormio, L., De Siati, M., Lorusso, F., Selvaggio, O., Mirabella, L., Sanguedolce, F., & Carrieri, G. (2011). Oral L-citrulline supplementation improves erection hardness in men with mild erectile dysfunction. Urology, 77(1), 119-122.

27. Esposito, K., Ciotola, M., Giugliano, F., Maiorino, M. I., Autorino, R., De Sio, M., ... & Giugliano, D. (2010). Effects of intensive lifestyle changes on erectile dysfunction in men. Journal of Sexual Medicine, 7(6), 2201-2208.

28. Estruch, R., Ros, E., Salas-Salvadó, J., Covas, M. I., Corella, D., Arós, F., ... & Martínez-González, M. A. (2013). Primary prevention of cardiovascular disease with a Mediterranean diet. New England Journal of Medicine, 368(14), 1279-1290.

29. Kapil, V., Khambata, R. S., Robertson, A., Caulfield, M. J., & Ahluwalia, A. (2015). Dietary nitrate provides sustained blood pressure lowering in hypertensive patients. Hypertension, 65(2), 320-327.

30. Konstantinidis, C., Tzitzika, M., Bantis, A., Nikolia, A., Samarinas, M., Kratiras, Z., ... & Skriapas, K. (2019). Female sexual dysfunction among Greek women with multiple sclerosis: Correlations with organic and psychological factors. Sexual Medicine, 7(1), 19-25.

31. Swan, S. H. (2021). Count down: How our modern world is threatening sperm counts, altering male and female reproductive development, and imperiling the future of the human race. Scribner.

32. West, S. G., McIntyre, M. D., Piotrowski, M. J., Poupin, N., Miller, D. L., Preston, A. G., ... & Skulas-Ray, A. C. (2014). Effects of dark chocolate and cocoa consumption on endothelial function and arterial stiffness in overweight adults. British Journal of Nutrition, 111(4), 653-661.

33. Budweiser, S., Enderlein, S., Jörres, R. A., Hitzl, A. P., Wieland, W. F., Pfeifer, M., & Arzt, M. (2009). Sleep apnea is an independent correlate of erectile and sexual

dysfunction. Journal of Sexual Medicine, 10(11), 2731-2739.

34. Leproult, R., & Van Cauter, E. (2011). Effect of 1 week of sleep restriction on testosterone levels in young healthy men. JAMA, 305(21), 2173-2174.
35. Brown, B. (2012). Daring greatly: How the courage to be vulnerable transforms the way we live, love, parent, and lead. Gotham Books.
36. Gottman, J., & Silver, N. (2015). The seven principles for making marriage work: A practical guide from the country's foremost relationship expert. Harmony Books.
37. Hatfield, E., Cacioppo, J. T., & Rapson, R. L. (1994). Emotional contagion: Studies in emotion and social interaction. Cambridge University Press.
38. Masters, W. H., & Johnson, V. E. (1970). Human sexual inadequacy. Little, Brown and Company.
39. McCarthy, B., & Wald, L. M. (2013). Mindfulness and good enough sex. Sexual and Relationship Therapy, 28(1-2), 39-47.
40. Weiner & Constance Avery-Clark (Routledge, 2017). Sensate focus in sex therapy: The illustrated manual. Routledge.
41. Althof, S. E. (2014). Treatment of rapid ejaculation: Psychotherapy, pharmacotherapy, and combined therapy. In Y. M. Binik & K. S. K. Hall (Eds.), Principles and practice of sex therapy (5th ed., pp. 112-137). Guilford Press.
42. Ventus, D., Gunst, A., Kärnä, A., & Jern, P. (2020). No evidence for long-term therapeutic effect of the stop-start technique for premature ejaculation: A randomized controlled clinical trial. Sexual Medicine, 8(3), 401-409.
43. Rastrelli, G., & Maggi, M. (2017). Erectile dysfunction in fit and healthy young men: Psychological or pathological? Translational Andrology and Urology, 6(1), 79-90.
44. American Association of Sexuality Educators, Counselors and Therapists (AASECT). (2023). AASECT

certified sexuality professionals. Retrieved from
AASECT website.

45. Gottman, J. M., & Gottman, J. S. (2017). The natural
principles of love. Journal of Family Theory & Review,
9(1), 7-26.

46. Nagoski, E. (2015). Come as you are: The surprising
new science that will transform your sex life. Simon &
Schuster.

47. Perel, E. (2006). Mating in captivity: Unlocking erotic
intelligence. Harper.

48. Sapolsky, R. M. (2004). Why zebras don't get ulcers: The
acclaimed guide to stress, stress-related diseases, and
coping. Henry Holt and Company.

49. Van der Kolk, B. A. (2014). The body keeps the score:
Brain, mind, and body in the healing of trauma. Viking.

50. Zilbergeld, B. (1999). The new male sexuality: The truth
about men, sex, and pleasure. Bantam Books.